# Saigon Siren

Copyright © 2024 Antonio Iannella.

All rights reserved.
No part of this publication may be reproduced, distributed, or transmitted in any form or by any means, including photocopying, recording, or other electronic or mechanical methods, without the prior written permission of the publisher, except in the case of brief quotations embodied in critical reviews and certain other non-commercial uses permitted by copyright law. For permission requests, write to the publisher/author, contact details
via website address below.

Australian Copyright Act 1968.

ISBNs
Paperback: 978-1-7636709-0-7
Hardcover: 978-1-7636709-1-4
eBook: 978-1-7636709-2-1

For privacy reasons, some names, locations, and dates may have been changed.
Manuscript editing by Cleo Miele.
Front cover art by Antonio Iannella.

First printing edition 2024.

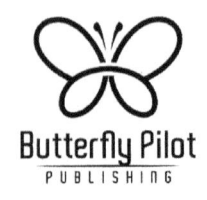

Butterfly Pilot
PUBLISHING

www.antonioiannella.com.au

# Contents

Prologue
    *Line in the Sand* ................................................................... *1*

One
    *Saigon Siren* ...................................................................... *5*

Two
    *Lemon Trees* .................................................................... *11*

Three
    *French Revolution* ........................................................... *17*

Four
    *Rock Paper Scissors* ........................................................ *22*

Five
    *Royal Melbourne Rowing Team* .................................... *30*

Six
    *The Dungeon* ................................................................... *40*

Seven
    *Mamma Mia* ..................................................................... *48*

Eight
    *Bystander* ......................................................................... *60*

Nine
    *Duke of Earl* ..................................................................... *67*

Ten
    *The Dungeon – Part Two* ................................................ *79*

Eleven
    *BS Period* ......................................................................... *91*

Twelve
    *The Girl in the Picture* .................................................. *104*

Thirteen
    *The Severing* .................................................................116
Fourteen
    *Happy Feet* ................................................................. 126
Fifteen
    *Six-String Heartache*.................................................131
Sixteen
    *Perfect Blue Buildings* ............................................. 142
Seventeen
    *The Interview*............................................................157
Eighteen
    *Cotton Candy* ........................................................... 166
Nineteen
    *Tell Him He's Dreaming*........................................... 179
Twenty
    *Neil Armstrong* .........................................................190
Twenty-One
    *Conspiring Universe*.................................................202
Twenty-Two
    *D-Day*........................................................................ 217
Twenty-Three
    *The Lion Tamers*.......................................................230
Twenty-Four
    *Lucky*.........................................................................248

Acknowledgements

PROLOGUE
# Line in the Sand

'Stroke? But you're so young!'
I often heard that at the beginning of my recovery. Even thought it myself at first—*What the ...? But I'm only thirty-eight!* In my brain's infinite wisdom, it decided to have its stroke while I was travelling through Vietnam with my three young daughters and their mother, leaving me paralysed from the neck down. Talk about pulling the rug out from beneath you, bursting your holiday bubble, squashing that travel bug—you get the picture.

There we were on an adventure of a lifetime, six months in planning and several weeks of learning to say 'thank you' in Vietnamese—'cảm ơn'. Organising a holiday takes longer than the holiday itself, but we often don't remember that bit. Our mind wipes it from our thoughts, deletes it from our files. In this case, it was our family holiday that was almost entirely erased from our memories.

A near-death experience is likely to overshadow tales about cruising across the muddy waters of the Mekong River, after all, or walking through fields that once staged a horrendous war. One moment I was listening to the tour guide talk about how the Viet Cong ambushed the American soldiers and the next, shortly after, I was lying in an Intensive Care Unit beneath fluorescent lights, listening to doctors speak about stroke.

Stroke is such an unglamorous name, but then I guess there's nothing glamorous about it; it just takes possession of you. I was a complete stroke novice before it happened to me. Suddenly, I was thrust into a world of needle jabs, oxygen masks and medical terms I couldn't spell.

One of the things I immediately learnt, through *firsthand experience*, was that stroke doesn't only happen to old people. In fact, it's reported that even babies in utero have suffered from this awful disease.

My only prior understanding of stroke was that it's caused by a blood clot that travels to the brain. This, I knew, as my mother had once had a minor stroke.

After the initial shock of almost dying in a foreign country, I made some decisions. Firstly, I wanted to understand what the hell happened and learn about this illness, what caused it, how it affects your body and, most importantly, how to fix it.

In particular, I recall the feeling of *What do I have to do to get back to normal?* I was practically rubbing my hands together, thinking, *Bring it on, I can do it. It might take me a year or so, but then I'm done. Next challenge, please!* Little did I know, my debilitating condition would consume my whole life and the lives of my loved ones around me.

Secondly, I decided I wasn't going to let stroke consume me. I'd just get on with it—battle through.

Writing this story felt like a natural progression. Having been a musician/songwriter for over twenty years, I often thought about writing stories, and now I had my own real-life tale to tell.

I eagerly began writing about my experience in the shape of a book. When I arrived at thirty thousand words, I came to a grinding halt. Almost head-butting my laptop screen, I quickly realised—with the help of others—that in all those pages, I hadn't even mentioned the word 'stroke'!

So, there it is, the very first word of my story in all its glory. Six tiny little letters making one HUGE word that gate-crashed my life in a boisterous Vince Vaughn fashion. I had been so caught up marvelling about the past, I'd navigated away from the present. Like the great Bono from U2 once said, 'We glorify the past when the future is grim,' or something like that. It's summed up perfectly in the book *The Power of Now:* 'The past gives us identity, the future brings us fulfilment, but we rarely live in the now.'

I've always been attracted to things slightly unique, offbeat, not so obvious. The one amongst mates who preferred to watch a Robert De Niro/Martin Scorsese film rather than a Spielberg blockbuster. The one who loved track nine on Radiohead's *OK Computer* rather than their hit single. The one who drove a classic 1963 Falcon—three-speed on the column—rather than a new Commodore. I have always searched for life's beautiful abnormalities, loved things slightly worn around the edges.

During my recovery, however, the thing I longed for, craved, and desired most was ... normality. Things like my old nine-to-five job, washing the dishes after dinner, walking up three steps without having to hold on to the rail, being able to open the jam jar without pressing it against my chest.

A stack of years into my recovery—I still refer to it as 'my recovery'—I have started to question it: When does a recovery period end? Is it when you are fully recovered? When you're satisfied with where you've reached? Or is it when you just stop trying? The truth is, I don't know. I still search for 'get better' exercise techniques. Still do my home physiotherapy routine, read biology books about the brain and go for regular walks trying to improve my stride, hoping the flashing sign above my head broadcasting 'MAN WITH DISABILITY' fades as I trundle through a busy shopping centre.

A quick thought: I'd vote for a political party that introduced a policy giving people who have been through the wringer like I have a Gold Pass—something that excuses you from life's daily annoyances and expenses. Police pull you over—'Excuse me, driver, do you know you changed lanes without indicating?' Gold Pass. Have to fill up your car at the petrol station? Gold Pass. Car rego due? Gold Pass. I'm sure you get the drift.

Okay, okay, so that's probably not going to happen. In the meantime, I guess I'll look out for four-cent savings on raw sugar.

Language warning! I don't often swear, but #@$%, after what I've been through, I think I've earnt it. Sitting silently in front of my laptop, I type with my one good hand: my right. My fingers don't have to stretch very far across the keyboard to write that particular expletive—*F* and *C* are just above each other and the *K* is only four keys to the right, the *U* just above the *K*. Easy.

Some people talk about the defining moment in their lives, a period that changed them forever, like watching the birth of their firstborn or graduating from university. My stroke was the line in the sand, the before and after. My own personal BC/AD (before Christ/after death)—or, as I have called it, BS/AS (before stroke/after stroke).

Through the following pages, I wish to expose you to not only the unpleasantness of stroke—the embarrassing and frustrating stories you never hear, the highs and lows, the heartache and pain—but also, hopefully, to the humorous side, and the incredible strengths of human kindness.

ONE

# Saigon Siren

My palms tingled, and my eardrums rumbled. Odd, but I didn't give it too much thought. Little did I know it was an early warning—a preview to the main feature where I played the leading role and my family, supporting roles.

I grabbed our bags and stepped off the hot, sweaty bus into the face of a typical humid Vietnamese midmorning. After purchasing our tickets, I proceeded to enter the grounds with my family. 'Here we are, about to enter underground tunnels built during the war ...' I reported while filming, unknowingly capturing the last few steps I would ever take as an able man. The line in the sand was about to be crossed.

The gate attendee ripped our tickets in half and directed us towards a shelter to watch footage of the Vietnam War, or, as the Vietnamese like to call it, the American War. We entered the open structure and sidestepped through rows of seated people to find some empty seats four pews back from the large suspended video screen.

'Hi! Has everyone commented on how crazy you are for travelling in Vietnam with such a young family?' a young Aussie mum seated behind us asked, crouched forward.

'Hi. Yes, you're right, they have. Where're you from?'

'We're from Brisbane. How about you guys?'

'Melbourne. What do you think of Vietnam?'

Like a transmitter radio losing reception, the conversation coming through in waves.

'I need to get some air,' I interrupted, stood, excused myself and headed for the exit.

The source of my physical abduction had begun its invasion.

I stepped out from beneath the shelter onto the patchy grass. I bent forward, placed my hands on my knees, the ground shifting and swaying as though I were on a small boat in a turbulent sea.

Full of her usual joy, my five-year-old daughter appeared in front of me.

'Molly, I don't feel well.'

'Yeah, yesterday my ears hurt,' she replied in her squeaky young voice, so innocent, so cute. I'll never forget that reply.

'Go get your mum.'

I looked up, shook my head to try gain some clarity, and my eyes bounced around like balls in a pinball machine. A nearby tree became two; my hands turned into four.

Molly returned with her mum. 'Are you ok?' fretted Silv. 'What's the matter?'

'I feel weak!'

Our tour guide, Chister, rushed over and placed his arm around my torso, aiding me to stand. 'What's wrong, mate?'

'Don't know ... I feel weak.' With my right arm over his shoulder, I leant on him like a crutch.

Pinned between them, struggling to contain my weight, Chister and Silv walked me across to the nearby first aid bay. As Chister rolled my arm off his shoulder and lowered me into a chair, the panic started setting in.

The commotion must have drawn attention; curious onlookers surrounded me, including the young Aussie mum with her family, their presence strangely comforting. I sat with my left elbow perched on a small table beside me, head buried in my hand, trying to disengage from my spinning surroundings.

I felt a palm rest on my forehead and a gentle grip squeeze my wrist as the first aid nurse timed my pulse against the seconds of his wristwatch. My heart pounding in rhythm with my rapid breaths, any words that entered my eardrums became wrapped with abrasive vibrations, my audible perception shifted.

In complete desperation, I managed to tell the nurse about my insect bite, swollen and visible on my bare left foot. A few days prior I had read a passage of text from my *Lonely Planet* guidebook describing similar symptoms as to what I was experiencing, a disease known as Breakbone Fever. We had had a marvellous day yesterday boating through canals of rice fields along the glorious Mekong River, visiting small rural farming villages and immersing ourselves in their brilliant, humble culture. It was there that I was bitten.

I clung on to this knowledge as some sort of feeble explanation. *It's just a bad reaction to the bite,* I told myself.

'Is he okay?' random unrecognisable voices asked.

Suddenly, a tidal wave of intense pins and needles washed over me, firing like a million tiny jackhammers penetrating my skin. It began in my left foot, crawled up my leg and buckled my knee. My elbow furiously collapsed off the table, and my head dropped hard against my chest. The sensation crossed my body and descended down my right side. Like an unwelcomed thief, it took possession.

I lost all composure, my body turned to jelly. Unable to hold myself up, the nurse was the only thing that prevented me from falling off the chair. That rumble in my eardrums I'd first heard before stepping off the bus had become consistent, increasing to distortion.

Like an out-of-focus camera, my vision blurred. I lost sight of my family standing right in front of me. I could hear the panic in everyone's voices.

That was it—the exact moment.

The defining event.

The precise point I crossed the line in the sand. A long chapter had just closed, and a new life-shattering one began.

'Silv, I can't see. Everything's gone blurry.' That realisation scared the crap out of me. *What the hell's happening?*

I felt my body lean forward. Several hands clasped under my arms and waist. They quickly decided to rush me to a local hospital. I was carried—or rather dragged—facedown across the harsh gravel surface that once was the battleground of a bloody war—*the American War*. The tops of my toes scraped a trail into the path, my nose a foot from the ground. I was being dragged like a wounded soldier.

Pulling, lifting, and handling me like a heavy sack of sand, an unmanageable weight, Chister, the Aussie mum's husband and the first aid nurse struggled to get me on board the tour bus. I wasn't able to assist whatsoever; my body dangled out of my control, as if it were a puppet with severed strings. I was slumped into a seat by the door, conscious, but my mind was completely detached from my body, petrified. I didn't know where my family was. Were they safe? I couldn't see them, couldn't hear them, and couldn't move to find them.

I don't recall the trip to the hospital, which I later learnt was a basic rural medical clinic. I don't know how long it took, but it felt like hours, forever. Many helpful hands lifted my sack sand body onto a stretcher, *an unmanageable weight*. Lying on my back, I saw the blue sky blur above as I was rolled from the bus into the medical clinic.

Strength abandoned, my hearing distorted and vision blurred, surprisingly I was still able to think okay and, with a slur, still somehow able to speak. 'I've been bitten, I've been … something bit me,' I murmured, the strained, cloudy words just able to stumble from my lips.

Riveted to the stretcher, I was strapped to the mattress in what appeared to be the foyer of the clinic. Light streamed in from the entry doors, or in from somewhere; I can't be sure. Silhouettes of bodies circled my bed, blurred outlines desperate to work out what was wrong, examining my feet, the insect bite, shining light into my eyes, assessing my blood pressure, heart rate. Banter and confusion bounced between the puzzled doctors, gibberish, mumblings, unconceivable words in an unrecognisable tongue. *Panic in everyone's voices.*

I could hear Silv in the background, faint and distant like a television on in the next room. Stressing her concern, voicing her alarm as the nurses yanked on her arm, pushing, pulling her aside, insisting she sign some sort of consent forms, wanting to see our passports. Hopeless hand gestures, broken English, desperate and deliberate. 'He's had a stroke,' she insisted. *'STROKE!'* The doctors blankly watched, message not received nor understood.

Chister was still with us amongst the madness, keeping an eye on the girls, attempting to calm the confusion, translating Silv's feared diagnosis.

I drifted in and out of consciousness. I was asked random questions to help keep me awake, but all I wanted was to float off into oblivion, fall deeper into myself. I only caught glimpses of the chaos. In a short blank spell, I found myself in another room, clothes stripped with a thin blanket covering me.

Silv stood by my side, caressing my forehead, calm and gentle. 'It's okay, just rest.' I wasn't able to move, couldn't feel my body. I was completely paralysed.

At some point an ambulance was ready to rush us back to Ho Chi Minh City, once named Saigon. My distorted hearing messed with my mind, taunted my perception. I could hear large trucks or planes rushing by. 'Are we near the airport?' I mumbled to Silv.

'Shhh, just rest. It's quiet here; there's no noise.' she remained brave.

'Where's the girls?'

'Don't worry, they're okay.' They sat a short distance from my bed. Charlotte fed little Maddie her milk while Molly sat quietly. Speaking then became difficult.

We were ninety minutes northeast of Vietnam's biggest city in a small village called Củ Chi, known for its seventy-five miles of underground war tunnels the Vietnamese had burrowed to ambush American soldiers during the war.

They rolled me back through the hectic light-filled foyer and out into the daylight, beneath the blurred blue sky and into the back of an ambulance. The paramedic placed an oxygen mask over my face. I took long, nervous breaths, holding on to myself, keeping still, resisting the urge to fall deeper, further and further away.

Charlotte and Molly sat in front, silent, consumed with fear. There weren't any seat belts.

I hadn't heard a sound from them and could only assume, could only hope, they were safe. Their silence said it all.

Silv squeezed precious ten-month-old Madeleine in her arms while seated beside my stretcher bed. Our baby girl's tiny limbs dangled from her mum's strong embrace.

Even though my vision was a blur, I could still see the distress on Silv's pretty face.

I was completely oblivious to the frightening one-and-a-half-hour ride to the manic city, the ambulance dodging, darting, weaving, and overtaking traffic at outrageous speeds in a frantic attempt to get me there ASAP. I don't recall even hearing a siren. I was tossed from one side of the stretcher to the other. My vague memory depicts the ambulance as an old transit van one may have used as a courier with very primitive medical gear, just enough to keep a patient alive.

We arrived frightened but safe at Saigon Hospital, only to find they weren't able to accommodate me. We took a further thirty-minute trip across the city to Franco Vasco Hospital.

There, I was disembarked from the ambulance, wheeled into the hospital, greeted by French doctors, and rushed through for an immediate MRI.

TWO

# Lemon Trees

I don't know what Silv said to relay the horrific news back to my family at home, nor do I really want to know. Just the thought alone makes my heart wrench, my throat swell and my eyes well up. I can only imagine how difficult it would have been for her to speak those painful words and how heartbreaking it must have felt for my family on the other end to hear them.

It was confirmed: the MRI revealed a stroke. Coincidentally, a leading international neurosurgeon was working at the hospital at the time. 'He has had a haemorrhagic stroke in the base of his brain,' he advised Silv, 'an inoperable location!'

With the end of his pen, the ICU's (Intensive Care Unit) head doctor scraped the bottom of my feet. 'Can you feel that?'

'No.' I was only able to speak a few words—*gibberish, mumblings.*

'You're very lucky, Mr. Iannella. If you have another stroke, you could ...' He paused. 'The next seventy-two-hours are critical.' *Rest and keep still. Try not to stress,* I was told.

The nurse hooked me up to the ICU heart monitor, sticking wired patches onto my chest. The steady pulse of the beep resonated through the sterile room, promising support my body wasn't able to provide.

I lay limp, fragile, all my senses suffocated. Strangled. Hushed, slurred words were all I could expel, almost unable to hear myself speak over the rumbling distortion in my ears. My vision met with a wall of blur, objects within the room appearing hazy, fragmented, pixelated. Fluorescent light interrupted by the cloudy shape of the nurse as she placed the breathing aid into my mouth, pressing it down against my tongue. Force-fed oxygen filled my lungs.

An intravenous line was inserted into the wrist of my right arm. The nurse suspended the fluid bag from its frame, and gravity delivered the medication down through the clear tube and into my veins. I don't know what the medication was; I just allowed the nurse to do what was required, what was needed. Resigned in fear and shock, I was at the mercy of these medical professionals as I lay in that bed in a foreign country, numb and silent, in an intensive care unit somewhere in the middle of Saigon.

I'd scan the room in an attempt to become familiar with my stale surroundings, squinting to make things clearer, but nothing changed; my eyes unable to make sense of my fragmented vision. Breathing slowly, in, out, in, out. 'The girls … the girls—where are the girls?' Silv was standing by my bed.

'It's okay, they're safe. Don't worry about them. Just rest.' I could just recognise her by the shape of her silhouette.

'Silv, I'm scared.'

I must have slipped into a lull of consciousness, still awake but disconnected from my surroundings. Kind of like that drowsy period just before you fall asleep, the state of being awake yet dreaming. My room was dim, silent, *sterile*. Silv had left.

Visiting times while I was in intensive care were very short. I only saw the girls briefly and could only imagine how afraid they must have felt. Their heads would pop up above the end of my bed. Silv had to pick them up and raise them over the bedrail so they could give me a peck on the forehead.

I assumed it was late in the evening, but I wasn't exactly sure. Other than the nonexistent aeroplanes and trucks whizzing by in my head, messing with my brain, the ward seemed still, quiet, empty.

A stranger entered my room and introduced himself. I don't recall his name, but he told me he was a friend of someone I knew back home in Melbourne and assured me he would do everything in his power to make sure I was okay.

He gave me hope—hope of rescue, salvage. *Get me out of here.* As desperate as I was, he could have told me he was Superman and said he was going to fly me home on his back and I would have believed him. So insecure, so vulnerable, so in need of answers, a reason, or help from anyone, someone, whoever—the tea lady, the floor sweeper, nurses, doctors. *Can anyone tell me, anyone, what the hell's going on?* Sure enough, Superman disappeared; I never saw him again.

Getting sleep was extremely difficult. It felt impossible. The stroke had caused my right eyelid to permanently remain sprung open. Wide. Wired. Unable to blink. My body was screaming out for some rest, longing to shut down. To retreat to the only place left I could turn to for some peace, to find some refuge and escape reality.

I lay awake for hours staring at the blurred ceiling, thinking yet not thinking, numb, nervous, and anxious, there but not there. It all went round and round in my head, trapped within my own mind, over and over again—*numb, nervous, anxious*—to the point of exhaustion until at last my pinned-open eye glazed over, stopped registering vision, and I was able to sleep.

In my waking hours there was problem after problem. The fluids being pumped into my veins made me desperate to urinate, but guess what—I couldn't. I didn't have the ability to conduct even that basic function that all living creatures relish daily. It wasn't possible. No matter how hard I tried, how hard I pushed, it just wouldn't come out.

It became painful, unbearable, as I felt like my bladder was about to explode. The pain grew excruciating; I began moaning and groaning, twisting and turning. The nurse came rushing in and frantically began fussing around, leaning over the bedrail at my waist, bed covers stripped to my ankles. I made all sorts of strange sounds, squirming in pain. I felt like I was about to give birth as I waited helplessly for the nurse to do something, anything. I could sense her panic, felt her frenzy as she fumbled about. I don't know what she was doing down there; I couldn't see, feel or hear.

Then suddenly, an incredible sense of relief washed over me. *Aaaahhh*—a feeling like no other, a moment of freedom, an *unmanageable weight* lifted, the pressure finally released. The pandemonium settled. Quietness returned and attached to my body was a catheter. *Phew!*

You may have heard the expression blokes use when drinking with mates: 'Don't want to break the seal.' From that moment on, I was like the Fountain of Trevi, like Niagara Falls, a raging river. Just as fast as the fluids entered my body, they also left. I filled bag after bag, enough fluid to fertilize an orchard of lemon trees.

With the breathing apparatus placed firmly in my mouth, aiding me to take slow, repetitive, and deliberate breaths, day two in the ICU came with the unpleasant discovery of not being able to swallow. I'd lost that ability, too.

The doctors feared phlegm could block my airflow, potentially choking me, which required the nurses to jam a suction hose into the back of my throat and vacuum up the unwanted mess like a seventies shag pile carpet. Backed up and going nowhere, a Monday morning rush-hour phlegm jam causing havoc in the back of my throat. It became very uncomfortable, not to mention dangerous, but the suction was far more painful, wrenching, agonising. My throat was so, so sore and tender, raw like a prime slice of scotch fillet.

During the evacuation my jaw would clench down tight, almost biting the end of the vacuum tube off. The suction process felt like it went on for way too long. *What's she doing in there, clearing a forest?* It left my throat feeling like it'd been scrubbed with a wire brush and turpentine.

Silv advised me that my brother Rem was flying over and should arrive by the following day. The news gave me a little lift. *That's it ... that's what I need. My little brother will save the day.*

Again, I got a quick close-up view of my daughters puzzled little faces as they reached over for an affectionate kiss. I just wanted to hold them, wrap my arms around them, protect them and protect me—protect *us*. Though they weren't really allowed into the ICU, the doc felt a short visit each day would lift my spirits. I often wondered, whilst blankly staring at the ceiling, what was going through their young minds and how Silv would have explained what had happened. From an adventurous holiday to watching their father all wired up to a machine, barely recognizable, pale and sad in this sombre environment. It was all incredibly difficult even for me to grasp; surely, they were struggling to keep it together.

Having a hinged-open right eyelid also ran the risk of my eyeball drying out. So, they began to administer eye drops to lubricate it. A great idea! However, this didn't solve my 'sleeping with one eye open' problem—at least there was no chance of anyone sneaking into my room to steal my wallet while I slept. They decided to tape my eyelid shut, which was a much-welcomed relief. Rather than attempting to slip into that awakened dream state, waiting for my eye to glaze over and stop registering vision—which was generally preceded with hours of blank staring and racing thoughts to the point of numbness—finally I was able to get some much-needed sleep, the first normal thing I regained.

Day two in the ICU was long, quiet, and painful. Despite my present physical state, my thinking process, once the cloudiness settled, faired best after my stroke. Strange, that. I desperately tried not to backtrack over the proceedings, but I guess it was inevitable. I traced through each of our steps the days leading up to my collapse: what I had eaten, how I had felt, if there any little sign. Now that my feeble insect bite theory had no footing and the doctors hadn't really elaborated as to why it had happened—not yet, anyway—I scrambled through my memory like an internet search engine scanning the web, a detective reassembling the evidence for a cold case.

The only thing I thought could possibly relate to my stroke was a headache I'd had several days prior. But it just didn't equate; it couldn't be that simple. I wasn't stressed or anything—*Christ! We were on holiday.*

Though my thought process was raw but still intact, my emotional state was a messy, overly abundant stir-fried banquet. The overwhelming urge to break down and cry stifled by the inability to produce tears. It was all going on in my head like a silent movie, throttled by the disablement of words, exhausted by the absence of energy. A monotonous spinning cycle of haunting thoughts, images, and visions interrupted with regular intermissions of nothingness, emptiness, vast and hollow fear. But all those crazy stir-fried emotions didn't translate on the outside. My blank, sunken composure hazardously disguised it all as I lay silent, listening to the reliable beep of the heart monitor.

'I want to go home,' I desperately muttered to Silv, nervous about the care I would receive in that foreign hospital. Afraid of dying in a strange country. Worried for the safety of my girls. I already had multiple needle punctures in my arm from failed attempts to insert the intravenous line into a vein. My wrist was battered and bruised from the barrage of injections by the duty nurses.

Silv immediately began her long, hard, and frustrating quest to get us home.

*Hang in there ... hang in there ... hang in there.*

THREE
# French Revolution

Although it was never said, Rem's biggest fear at that time was coming over to Vietnam to bring his brother back home in a body bag. He arrived with a long list of well wishes, love, and adoration. Silv's desperate Facebook post had created a Mexican wave of panic and concern, spreading across family, friends, and colleagues like a wild bushfire at the height of a dry, desolate summer.

Emergency rescue, too far away.

It was just before the long Easter weekend of 2009. My stroke had arrived on a Thursday, April ninth, one day short of not-so-Good Friday, the line in the sand for Jesus. Most of Australia was preparing for four days of overeating amongst family members, drinking tawny port from tiny glasses and exchanging chocolate bunnies, while I lay in intensive care clinging to life.

The French Revolution (my ICU doctors) monitored me like they were guarding the borders of France. During his routine observation, Doctor Napoleon (head doc) discovered my immune system was under attack. The enemy was fast approaching, my defences compromised.

He unleashed the cavalry on the duty nurse.

'What are you doing?! You should be watching him!' he shouted. 'He could have another stroke and die, you silly woman!' I couldn't see the interrogation, and I wasn't able to hear every word, but his tone spoke volumes. His frustration was epic.

I had contracted pneumonia.

The doctors didn't know how or why it happened. It may have been the state of my vulnerable health, my body too weak to defend itself, or the permanent circulation of the air conditioner, allowing my body temperature to plummet, or maybe both. Who knows—it just meant danger! I was placed on seventy-two-hour life watch with hourly observations.

I'll never forget Doctor Napoleon's softly spoken words, 'You're just breathing enough to stay alive … good,' as he leant in and whispered into my ear.

The taped-shut eyelid idea seemed to do the trick. After a decent night's sleep, day three came with some small but promising improvements.

A feel-good surge filled my room. A buzz of energy flitted around, putting smiles on the Revolution's faces as they proudly watched me wiggle my right-hand fingers and toes. 'Well done, good, good.' Doc Napoleon's hand rested on my forearm, his French accent coloured with a hint of hope.

The doctors went to great lengths to care for us, doing whatever they could to help. Even in my depleted state, I was humbled to hear how Napoleon's wife had taken our girls out for an afternoon of swimming in their pool, sharing a warm sunny day with her own kids. The heartfelt gesture provided a tiny slither of relief, of gratitude. The silent movie I was constructing in my head showed them smiling, having fun, being children.

Although movement on my right side had increased and I could now scratch my own nose, press the nurse call button and desperately, lovingly, finally hold one of my daughters' tiny hands through the gaps of the bedrails, it still wasn't a gentle paddle across calm, clear waters. The seventy-two-hour critical lifeguard-watch period was nearing its end; however, choppy seas still posed a threat. My temperature rose and fell like a Gold Coast theme park ride.

With a limp, lifeless left side and an unreliable, limited right, with a combined capacity only capable of preventing my head from rolling off the bed, my body felt like it belonged to someone else.

An array of confusing sounds continued to reverberate in between my ears. There were strange noises hissing behind my forehead and fuzzing at my temples, a helicopter landing on my pillow, a propeller rotating, an engine revving—I thought I even heard Charlie Watts (RIP) bashing out Rolling Stones classics beside my bed. It freaked me out. I knew the intensive care room was dead silent, but in my head, trucks, buses, trains and aeroplanes charged through nonstop.

I couldn't work out where they were coming from. *What's that noise?* I'd ask myself, lying there in complete silence. *I can hear a beat ... is that a motorcycle?* It would flip from one noise to another but it was always on, full throttle. I felt distorted, marooned, and had no faith in my own thoughts, no dependence on my own body. I was wired to a machine, a breathing aid, a catheter. Throw blurred vision into the twisted melting pot of perception and my world only consisted of understanding things within a foot in front of me.

Easter Sunday painfully arrived, but there was no resurrection for me. Nonetheless, I did regain the simple task of swallowing. And you know what that meant? No more sucking my insides out, no more vacuuming that shag pile throat or clearing my forest of phlegm!

My right arm was riddled with punctures from the jabbing of needles; the hospital must have assigned the trainee nurse to practice on me. There weren't too many available veins left, so the head nurse had a crack at relocating the intravenous line into my neck. After her third attempt, she finally found a vein willing to cooperate.

For my entertainment, the staff wheeled in a portable television, propped it by my bed and set it to a local channel. I don't know what their thinking was behind that; all I could see was flashing light, the *hazy, fragmented, pixelated* images thickening the fog, stirring the confusion, pushing me deeper into myself. I couldn't bear to watch. It hurt to listen. The Vietnamese dialogue was disorientating, confusing. I was unsure if it was me who couldn't hear properly or if it was a foreign language. Well, the local language, rather; I was the foreigner.

Days and nights, nights and days overlapping, melding together. The sterile, sombre room didn't adhere to time; it set its own pace, played by its own rules. Just trying to express a few words was exhausting. I'm sure I slept a lot. I don't even recall seeing Silv, Rem or the kids at this point. All I had to carry me was a vague sense, a faint flicker in me that knew my brother was there, that knew my girls were waiting for Daddy to come home.

Sleeping was accompanied by some frightening nightmares. There were a few different reoccurring types. This is the one that haunted me most while in the ICU.

I was placed into a hospital laundry trolley, then transported down into the basement, wheeled through dusty abandoned corridors and into a dark underground room. Draped in surgical blues, a masked person stepped in close, their eyes wide open, bloodshot, fear riddled. They leant in over me, then attempted to remove my eyeballs.

On one occasion, while I was having that exact dream, a nurse woke me at the precise moment my eyeballs were being removed. In complete fear and in survival mode, I grabbed her by the wrist. With just enough strength in my right hand, I was able to push her away, fend her off. She had to calm me down, cool my theme park ride temperature and return me to ground zero. ICU normal, steady, sterile.

Those dreams continued for several weeks.

By that stage Silv was a few steps closer to coordinating my return home, her tiresome and relentless efforts finally finding a service to conduct a rescue flight.

The mission went a bit like this: Their assigned doctor would run some basic health tests, assess the information, and decide whether I was fit for a twelve-hour journey. If so, dates would be scheduled, payment for the service made and flights booked.

The doctor accompanied by a nurse would escort me to the airport via ambulance. Through special arrangements with airport officials, I'd be transferred onto the plane in a wheelchair and placed into a seat with the doctor and nurse seated on either side of me, monitoring my condition through the entire flight.

Once we arrived, an ambulance was to meet us on the tarmac at Melbourne Airport, which would then carry me across to Royal Melbourne Hospital. Crazy!

FOUR

# Rock Paper Scissors

My heart was racing, galloping through the ICU, down the lift and onto a lower floor. The new surroundings were confounding, too much to take in with its different noises, changed atmosphere. I felt lost, displaced, paranoid.

The room appeared to be at an odd shape, and I couldn't quite work out how my bed was positioned. *Am I butted up against the wall?* Questions, thoughts, and fears fuelled my vulnerability—*Or am I in the middle of the room?*—as I was plagued by minor, irrelevant, desperate needs.

It was a twin share, bright, basic. I didn't get the bed by the window, but I caught my first glimpse of glaring sunlight in six days.

The first few hours were spent blankly staring, gazing with empty eyes at the ceiling, trying to distinguish the different ceiling fixtures. *Is that an air vent or light fitting?* I was still only able to process things within one foot in front of me. Close.

The ward nurses were all quite young and relaxed in their approach, leisurely. With their grasp of the English language—three steps behind the ICU team's—and my vocab on a forced sabbatical, communication was difficult. If I asked for a sip of water, they'd fluff my pillow; if I asked them to fluff my pillow, they'd give me a sip of water. It was confusing, almost comical. It felt like satire.

My right-side function continued to take micro steps forward. The clenched numbness my body felt had turned down a notch, revealing an odd, permanent, and prominent pins-and-needles sensation, *a million tiny jackhammers on overdrive,* beneath my skin. Like the aftereffect of a limb falling asleep multiplied by a thousand, then shrink-wrapped in cling film. *Tight.*

Better still, I had regained some movement on my lifeless left side. I was just able to raise my arm off the bed, move my hand and bend my ankle. *Look at me go!* And though watching my fingers wiggle gave me a buzz, it also felt very bizarre, like it was someone else's hand moving. Weird!

The hospital physiotherapist had been in to see me, and while lying on my back, he gave me a few alternative exercises for each limb. Rotate my foot and wrist, bend my knee and elbow and do some leg raises.

Substituted for the catheter was an adult-sized diaper. Yes, you read that correctly ... a diaper. A nappy. But just hang on! There was method in their madness, some reasoning in their reason, but I'll get to that in a sec. What this also meant—the good bit—was that I could go *au naturel.*

Now that the Monday morning rush hour phlegm jam at the back of my throat had been given the all clear for traffic to flow and I could once again swallow, I had been spoon-fed soup for the last few days by the nurses. Whilst wearing a baby's bib, too, because my rubber-band lips couldn't stay closed tight enough to prevent the first non-liquid drip-fed meal I had eaten in almost a week from running down my chin—all of which meant the Revolution had new concerns.

I hadn't yet passed solids.

Wearing a diaper isn't as bad as you may think. It's quite a liberating feeling just peeing as you please, and it would be ideal at a barbecue. No need to excuse yourself to use the loo, and for the ladies, no long queues in nightclubs.

As I mentioned at the beginning, these are *the embarrassing and frustrating stories you never hear.* The next few paragraphs cover the lowest point of my physical condition—the most humiliating experience I have ever had. Ever! I deliberated over whether I should even disclose this incident, as it's not exactly my finest moment! But I promised to deliver *'the stories you never hear'*. So, if you have a weak stomach or you're planning to eat once you finish reading this section, I *strongly* suggest you skip the following few paragraphs. For your convenience, I have indicated with an asterisk (*) below where it's safe to continue from.

The male nurse must have lost at rock, paper, scissors, as he was the one assigned the challenging duty to conduct an enema on a severed-stringed puppet body of a man—me.

He first began by demonstrating, with charade gesturing, how he was going to lift me out of bed and into the wheelchair that had the seat cut out to replicate a toilet seat. Then he would wheel me into the bathroom, administer the enema and then back into bed.

*Sounds easy enough*, I thought.

He began by lowering the bed height, then raising the head end till I sat semi-upright. Leaning me forward and holding me steady, my right arm was placed over the back of his neck, replicating a reverse headlock wrestling position, as he shuffled my jalopy mannequin body towards the bed's edge. My legs unfolded over the side, numb feet dangling in the air.

With his braced arms lowered around my midsection like a rugby tackle, I was jackknifed off the bed and into the wheelchair, catapulted like a crash test dummy.

Safe landing.

I wasn't sure what exactly was supposed to happen during the enema. It was the first time I had ever had one, so I didn't know what to expect. But not much happened at all. I felt the exact same: *lousy!* A whole lot of fuss for a whole lot of nothing.

He fumbled me back into bed as the room was spinning, *swaying as though I were on a small boat in a turbulent sea*. I was awkwardly dressed in a fresh clean nappy and left to rest, crash test dummy exhausted.

Here comes the humiliating bit. It's not too late; you can still skip this section if you wish.

As I lay in bed, about an hour later, my stomach began to twist and turn.

I pressed the call button.

The nurse leisurely rushed in—far too leisurely for my liking!

It had begun. It was friggin' horrible, squirting out everywhere from all sides of my nappy, covering the bed sheet, running into the blanket, down my legs, up my belly. It was all over the place, and it smelt terrible and looked disgusting. It was like a sewerage plant had exploded in my diaper. It continued to pour out uncontrollably—it just wouldn't stop, and the nurse had to call for backup. I was so embarrassed, ashamed of myself.

*Oh my god.*

A team of nurses circled my bed, all cute young women witnessing my body excrete the buildup of soup. They wiped desperately, frantically, attempting to clean me up and strip my bed, trying to eradicate all evidence, trying to stay brave, unaffected. *They'll be scarred for life!* I couldn't believe what was happening. I had no control at all; my body doing what it liked, what it pleased, with a mind of its own. All I could do was watch and shamefully wait till it was finished.

*World, swallow me whole!*

And that, my friend, was—and still is—the absolute lowest I had ever reached in my entire life. At thirty-eight years old, I shat my nappy!

\* If you made the decision to skip the last section, here are a brief few words to describe what you missed: enema, explosion, and a massive clean-up mission!

'Hi, Antonio, how are you? I am Dr. So-and-So ... I will be escorting you on your rescue flight back to Australia.' My personal Captain America, confident, direct, here to save the day. 'But first, we need to do some observations on you.' He placed his palm gently on my forehead. 'I've been advised you have pneumonia.' He was standing close, within my one-foot visual range. Through his gold-framed glasses, he looked straight into my eyes. 'Well, we have to get that under control before we can fly anywhere.' Blond moustache, clean shaven, buttoned short-sleeve shirt, stocky.

Over the following days, with his superpowers, Captain America was to keep a close eye on me and monitor my condition. Once stable enough, he'd make the required arrangements for the long haul home. The danger of flying with an elevated body temperature could be catastrophic; they were concerned it may cause another stroke, but I wasn't too concerned about the danger. I was prepared to take a chance. All I wanted was to get out of there, get home and get better. I needed to feel safe, secure and have my family and friends around me. I needed to hear doctors and nurses speak to me in English, to help me to understand, to provide direction. A prognosis.

A sexy, seductive voice echoed from the doorway.

'Are you ready for your sponge bath, sir?'

There she stood, an extraordinary beauty. Long legs, long black hair, a short tight nurse's uniform. Stunning! She moved in close, reached over the bedrail, peeled the blanket back and sensually, delicately, gently unfastened the Velcro straps to my nappy—it was all I was wearing. She began sponging me down with poised lips, flawless porcelain skin. It was heaven. *Please don't stop*. I was so relaxed I was floating, melting into the mattress. She giggled; I smiled.

Although some of the generic medical procedures they conducted on me were, shall we say, less than impressive—such as the *barrage of needle jabs*—their TLC skills were second to none! And perhaps my imagination about this beauty bolted free, ran wild. I received warm, soothing sponge baths, they spoon-fed me soup, and they gave me sips of refreshing water and bathed my forehead with a cool cloth when my temperature was skyrocketing.

What was most impressive was how they changed my bed sheets without getting me out of bed by *jackknifing*. They would roll me to one side, then tuck the sheet beneath my body, and then roll me over to the other side of the bed to remove the sheet completely. I just kept still, as if I was mummified.

Our language barrier may have prevented us from communicating beyond basic levels of understanding, but I grew fond of these people. Their caring nature was humbling, grounding.

*The incredible strengths of human kindness.*

The ambulance came to a stop on the tarmac a short distance from the aeroplane. We were to wait for further instructions before boarding. Silv and the kids were to meet us on board, nervously waiting in the departure lounge.

Rem had already left a few days prior; he would have already been in Melbourne by that stage.

The few days leading up to our departure crept along at a snail's pace, excruciatingly. My body temperature escalated sharply, then dropped dramatically through the course of each day—I was still on the *Gold Coast theme park ride called Pneumonia*. Captain America had concerns about my yo-yoing internal climate, my boiling barometer. But he believed it was manageable; he had it under control. I had it under no control.

Anyhow, there was no turning back now. It was all in place. Signed, sealed, but yet not delivered. Eleven days had now passed since my life had taken a dramatic turn, since I had crossed that line. I couldn't wait to get home and see my family, my friends. Hug them, be hugged, hold them, be held. Get better. Start my recovery in an Australian hospital, where everyone spoke English.

The ambulance door swung open; we were ready to go. I was rolled out and immediately struck by the intensity of the heat, reminding me I was still in Vietnam. It was around midnight but the humidity still made the air thick, muddy, dense. Finding my breathing rhythm took time, effort.

I was switched from the stretcher to a wheelchair and lifted in between Captain America and the male nurse accompanying us on this harrowing journey. They pushed me along the tarmac and into a large freestanding elevator, a purpose-built lift for difficult situations like this one—emergencies. With no air it was baking hot, toasted by the all-day sun. The elevator moved upwards, stopped momentarily, and then the doors shifted open, revealing the aeroplane. A short suspended metal bridge linked the elevator to the plane's doors, canopied across the tarmac. My stomach was like a vice, tight, contracted. My jaw clenched as though I was biting off that phlegm jam suction hose. My emotions were raw, tender, *like a prime slice of scotch fillet*. I just wanted this thing to end. To stop.

Captain America pushed me across the canopied bridge. The volume of the tarmac activity was abrasive, punishing. The aeroplane's idling engines expelled a coarse heated draft that collided into my body, my face, overpowering the permanent distortion I heard in between my ears, silencing Charlie Watts's drumming. I was terrified!

Just as we boarded the empty plane, Captain America's mobile phone rang. It was Silv calling from the terminal lounge, asking if we were on board, 'Because we're not getting on that flight without him!' she said firmly.

Once again wedged between the two, they lifted me out of the wheelchair and into my seat. The nurse sat to my right and doc to my left, just over the aisle.

Out of the corner of my eye I could see shapes of boarding passengers, people searching for their seats and placing their bags in overhead compartments, goggling at me as they walked past. *What's happened to him?* I felt like an illuminated alien. A spectacle, a circus attraction. Paranoid.

A sense of calm washed over me once my family boarded the plane. My girls greeted me with affectionate hugs, kisses, and weary smiles, then headed to their seats.

The seat belts sign turned on. We were ready for take-off.

I don't recall much of the flight; the hot and cold flushes made time lapse, fade away. I don't remember the take-off or the landing. We sat in business class, the girls sitting back in economy. They would pop down for short visits, giving me *hugs, kisses, weary smiles.*

My yo-yoing temperature continued to wreak havoc, keeping the nurse on his toes during the entire course of the flight. His fashion of caring was remarkable, cooling me when I escalated sharply, then covering me when I dropped dramatically. Checking my vital signs on the hour, every hour. A timekeeper, a lifesaver, while Captain America took a break from fighting crime and saving the world by napping, snoring. Gold-framed glasses, stocky.

It was nice to hear the nurse talk about other things than stroke as he kept me from *drifting off to oblivion.* His English was three steps ahead of the ICU team's, and he spoke passionately about his loved ones at home, his children.

I couldn't thank him enough for the way he looked after me during that flight—he was *a lifesaver.* We parted with a warm embrace once we arrived in Melbourne.

Home sweet home.

It took some time to get me off the aeroplane, as all the passengers were required to disembark first. A cherry picker type of lift parked beside the plane's exit was used to lower me down to the tarmac, and the ambulance was there waiting.

Even in my depleted physical state, airport customs conducted their standard routine checks, making sure Captain America had all his paperwork in order.

A casual ambulance ride from airport to hospital and I already felt a little more at ease, comforted by the Aussie accents of the paramedics.

*G'day, mate.*

FIVE

# Royal Melbourne Rowing Team

In an attempt to determine whether I had all my marbles in line, the emergency doctor fired a series of questions at me.

'What's your name? When were you born? Do you know where you are? What day is it?' Like a Purana Taskforce interrogation.

He continued with a series of routine tests, probing, poking, squeezing, pulling, pushing. 'Can you feel this? Can you feel that?'

Function on my right side was steadily improving, sailing along—I could scratch my nose, press a button, hold something—with the new addition of raising a cup to my lips for a drink, albeit nervously. The doc's blunt needle point jabbing various places across my better right half were vague, dull, faint, washed out like a fading memory, while my persistent and disobedient left half refused to acknowledge any stimulation at all. Nothing. Still on vacation in Vietnam.

'I want you to push against the weight of my body.' He raised my left leg, bent it at the knee and placed the sole of my foot against his chest. 'Okay, push.' My knee wobbled, trembled, about to buckle like it had back at the tunnels in the first aid bay. A long minute passed with the doctor quietly standing there, slightly leaning forward, waiting for me to push him backwards. Waiting, my foot on his chest, him going nowhere as we sat in silence.

When I had first arrived at Royal Melbourne Hospital, straight after the ambulance chaffier ride from tarmac to emergency, I was placed in an empty small square holding room. There I waited for the emergency doctor to look me over, to conduct his Purana-like soft interrogation.

It was the first time I had been alone since my wardroom back in Vietnam. I finally had a moment to process it all: the Vietnamese midnight heat, the sun-baked elevator, the suspended metal bridge, the rescue flight, the cherry picker, the waiting ambulance. So heavy. The room was warm, too warm. I felt flushed, rosy-cheeked. My heart was full of dread, my head full of fog as I waited to be seen, to be healed, lying there in disbelief.

Time in that room stretched on for hours, or maybe it was only minutes. *Have they forgotten about me?* Through the opaque glass door, I could see blurs of people walking past—staff, nurses, doctors, ghostlike silhouettes. *Where is everyone?* Longing to see my family, wanting, needing to let go, to surrender my emotions, to feel safe. To be held.

When the opaque door rolled open and the doctor walked in, alone, my heart sank; it plummeted like my temperature. I wanted so badly to see my dad, my sisters, my brother, my girls. All of them.

'Okay, grab hold of my fingers.' The deep inquiry continued for twenty or so minutes more, but I desperately ached for it to end. I had nothing left in me; I was running on empty. It had only been a short while since we had landed, since I had been cherry picked from an aeroplane after twelve hours of riding the punishing Gold Coast theme park ride.

'Squeeze as hard as you can.' It was my very first attempt in the AS period—after stroke—that I had consciously used my left hand for anything other than wiggling my fingers or bending my wrist.

I wasn't emotionally ready to witness my hands' inability, couldn't bear to hazily watch the impaired function of my deformed fingers. It was too much too soon; I just didn't have the resolve. The strength tests went far beyond the basic exercises I had done at

Franco Vasco Hospital. My lead balloon arm wanted to recoil, fall to my side, and lay untouched upon the mattress. Detached, distant, disconnected.

The last few minutes were spent exploring my visual ability, the windows to my shattered soul. 'Follow my moving finger with your eyes,' he asked while pointing to the ceiling. 'Keep your head still.' This seemingly simple task was hopelessly challenging. My vision jittered, my eyes unable to keep track as a blurred trail followed his moving finger—*too much too soon*.

Finishing up his examination—the Purana Files—he determined where to send me, who was next in line to help. My final task was to produce a smile ... something I hadn't done a lot of lately!

Initially, immediately after my fall, as you know, I was paralysed from the neck down. After a few days or so, movement to my right began to return. However, above my neck was a different story. The paralysis was on the opposite side. My body was predominately affected on the left, and my head on the right. *Weird*. Which meant the left end of my smile curled upwards, as it should, but the right end made a sad, sloppy sunken smile, sort of going downwards. Deflated.

By the end of the examination, I felt like a pair of old ratty runners. My soul was worn out, falling apart. Retired. 'Someone will be with you shortly.' With that, the doctor left the room, giving me another quiet moment to take it all in, to rewatch the highlights from the silent movie in my head. Snapshots.

Dust from the past twenty-four hours was beginning to settle, subside. I began to feel more strange, odd, and awful new sensations surfacing across my body, rearing their ugly heads. My awareness was beginning to realign itself; my senses were awakening. My face felt tight, taunt, ready to rip, like cling film stretched across a bowl of leftovers, while a colony of bull ants seemingly feasting on my skin. My head felt like it was wrapped in a crown of thorns, a headlock. *One-foot vision, rubber-band lips, severed-string body, Charlie Watts.*

Here's a bit of a post-stroke 'bad to good' running order on my physical and emotional state.

Leading the race—well ahead of the pack, but not necessarily winning—was the left side of my body. The shrink-wrapped sensation was beginning to give a little. To execute movement—to wiggle my fingers or toes, bend my elbows and knees, or raise my arms and legs—required conscious thought, instructions. It wasn't *au naturel*. Commands to my affected left side were contaminated with a time lapse, a delay, a stutter; the message hesitated before arriving at its destination.

Coming in second, a strong contender, was my vision, blurry, slow, and cloudy. A contributing factor to my *'only understanding things that were within a foot in front of me'* syndrome.

And hot on its heels, a favourite paying good dividends, was my hearing, or lack of it. Confusing noises rattled around in my head nonstop. Sounds were harsh, distorted. Speech vibrated like it was spoken through a muzzle, and everyone was required to speak sssllllooowwweeerrr, *LOUDER* and stand closer.

Somewhere nestled in the pack, an outsider that had the potential to snatch the prize, all dressed in various distracting colours, was my dizziness, known by its peers as 'vertigo'. If I turned my head too quick, the room would spin in slow motion, showing smeared movement—*world, swallow me whole*. The best thing to do to combat this was to lie completely still, so that's what I did ... a lot!

Rounding up the pack, steady and reliable—coming in lucky last, but not necessarily losing—was the right side of my body. Its strength was good; the movement of my arm and hand, though restrained and shaky, was nearing normal. Strangely, though, the dull fading memory of a touch continued to further reveal numbness whilst at the same time exposing a contradicting heightened sensitivity wrapped in throbbing pins and needles from those *millions of tiny little jackhammers on overdrive*. Two polar opposite sensations: numbness and heightened sensitivity.

Every good horse race deserves spectators. Up on their feet cheering on all the competitors, placing bets with the bookies, losing a load, and cursing both the horse and rider was the state of my emotions. The vast variety of attendees at this exclusive event called My Stroke ranged from despair to fear, confusion, isolation, sadness, pain, uncertainty, and shock ... all there, all dressed to the nines, intoxicated, and behaving like imbeciles.

Most of the time, apart from the spells of overheating, the mechanics of my thought process was reasonably well oiled. I had many lengthy conversations with myself, a continuous internal monologue, till there was nothing worthwhile left to say. Then, I'd repeat it all over again. *What if this happens? What if ... ?*

Trying to transfer those conversations, thoughts and questions into actual real words—words that left my lips and that others could hear, understand—required an energy that wasn't readily available. No matter how hard I revved my engine, my gearbox was stuck in neutral, and I had no traction to produce audible dialogue.

Finally, my longing was relieved. My emotions surrendered, let go. I could feel safe and be held. My family were allowed in to see me. Breaking through the dam's wall, my tears released themselves, the first since collapsing. Falling. Flooding. My dad, sisters Carmel and Ange, brother Rem, Silv and our girls were all there, all together. There wasn't much they could say or do besides sob in each other's arms and mutter words like *Are you okay? How do you feel? I love you.*

The last time we were all in a hospital room together, heartbroken, was when our mother had suddenly passed away. She was rushed to hospital, but they couldn't save her. We all got there too late to say our last goodbyes. The spirit had already left her body.

Whenever I have a flashback, a *snapshot* of my time in hospital, lying there in that empty small square holding room, paralysed, petrified and surrounded by my sobbing family, it still hurts. It still makes me emotional. I'm writing this section with tears in my eyes.

Losing a loved one under such crushing circumstances doesn't often happen to most of us, but yet there we were once again, reliving the same heartache as when Mum passed away. Dad has never been one to openly express his emotions, and though I wasn't able to clearly see the anguish on his face, I could feel his pain with astute clarity.

Their presence, the people I loved and cherished, gave me that safety I craved, the security I needed. For that half hour or so in a small room, a family stood united in the face of adversity, together, supportive. Light filtering in through the opaque glass door, closed to the outside world for our privacy, allowing us to grieve, cry and hug. A thirty-minute unification that will flicker in my heart for the rest of my life.

It was all I had thought I needed: my family by my side, finally. But not having answers to the how, why, and when of it all still left a gap, a hollowness. I felt like I was being steered into the unknown. Heading into darkness. When a nurse entered my room on a routine check, I wanted them to make me better. If a doctor asked me questions, I hoped for a quick fix solution.

It didn't take too long for me to work it out—to realise I *was* being steered into the unknown, into darkness, uncertainty. There was no fast track back to myself, no speedy 'get better' trick the nurse could conduct or the doctor could perform, no medication that would erase this nightmare.

The very first night in a ward, in Melbourne, my hometown, was disturbing. Those unsettling dreams continued, this one just as frightening as the eyeball removal attempt.

I dreamt I was at sea, asleep in a cabin on an old timber boat. Dull light flickered from the wall-mounted candelabras, dispersing random waves of eerie shadows. Above my bed head to the left was a small trap door. The trap door creaked open, and a queue of ghosts began to enter through the door, stepping over my shoulder and across my bed one by one in single file, ghost after ghost. There were so many of them, and the leader carried an old lantern. They were all dressed in drab, colourless period clothing from the thirties or forties that appeared wet, sea-soaked from the ocean.

I shot out from the nightmare and woke in a fright, sweating, boiling, panicked. Confused as to where I was, it seemed I was still in the middle of the dream, witnessing it, watching it unfold. Riveted to the bed as I was, the ghosts stepped over my left shoulder and across my body, stepping down off my mattress and exiting another door.

Once the ghosts all left, I pressed the call button, in a state. The nurse rushed in, not so leisurely this time! 'It's okay, you're safe.' She bathed my forehead, gave me sips of water. 'Just relax. You're home now.'

Being that it was my first night at Royal Melbourne Hospital, due to all the activity—doctor's examinations, nurse's checks, settling in, seeing family—I hadn't had much of a chance to blankly stare, to ceiling gaze and familiarize myself with my new surroundings. *Is that a light fitting, or air vent?*

The room was long and narrow. I don't know why, but it felt creepy. I shared the space with several others—three or four, maybe five; can't be sure. Only faint dimmed lighting was on while we slept, so when I woke in fright from the nightmare, I thought I was still on the boat, at sea. It took quite a bit of time for the nurse to settle me. She stood by my side for a little while, holding my hand.

The next morning, the hospital psychologist paid me a visit. 'You have been through a horrific traumatic experience,' she spoke gentle, calmly. 'Your mind is dealing with the turmoil during sleep.' Tears streamed down my cheeks. 'If the nightmares continue, try to visualize your favourite place, a time where you felt joy or happiness.'

Later that day, I made a mental shortlist in preparation of some of my favourite times and places. At the top of that list was picturing myself in Thailand, travelling, not a care in the world. Young, free. Blissful.

When the ward lights went out in the evening at ten, I fell asleep quite easily in minutes. Stroke sucked the living energy out of me, so losing valuable sleep and waking in a state of stress from a horrible nightmare would further zap my brain, making me close to catatonic.

Visualising Thailand, golden beaches, clear blue waters, *not a care in the world,* seemed to work. Slowly, the daunting dreams became less frequent, and eventually they stopped.

The Royal Melbourne Rowing Team—stroke ... rowing ... get it?—are a team of neurologists and neurosurgeons. 'The best in the state,' said one of the nurses.

'Hi, Antonio, how are you feeling?' I was first surprised by how young they all were. 'We're the hospital's neuro team.' Six of them circled my bed, a team of mixed genders and serious faces. 'Let's do some tests on you.' One of them did all the talking, the head doc, presumably, while the others scribbled down illegible notes.

Head Doc began by conducting what was to become the all-too-familiar observation routine, leaving out the soft interrogation; he most likely had already read the Purana Files.

Pinpricks to my feet, legs, arms, and face. Squeezing fingers and pushing against force. A dance routine that would have received a score of straight tens by the panel of judges on *Dancing with the Stars.*

They began to draw particular attention to my staggered eye movement. Stepping in closer, looking harder. 'Follow my finger with your eyes,' Head Doc would request while watching my trembling eyes stagger along, falling behind the moving finger, losing track.

It fascinated them; they were marvelled. *What have we got here?* Faces turned from serious to intrigued. *A perfect specimen for medical study.* Repeating the examination in different alternative variations, they directed me, *How many fingers am I holding? Tell me when you can see my hand. Which finger is this? Follow my finger. Follow the pen. Touch my finger, then touch your nose.* Far out ... what a head spin. I was just waiting for him to say *Pull my finger.*

'In a few days we'll get you to have another MRI,' said one of the other doctors, 2IC. 'This should allow enough time for the blood around the stroke to drain so we can get a clearer picture of the damaged area.' Finally, some answers. *When. How. Why!*

The initial MRI I'd had in Vietnam revealed a haemorrhagic stroke, but due to the build-up of blood, they weren't able to determine why it had happened. 'Once we get a better look, we can think about the next step and decide whether surgery is required or move straight onto rehabilitation.'

Although the doctors didn't elaborate as to why I may require surgery, they briefly mentioned—speaking slower, louder and standing closer—that the haemorrhage could have been the cause of an aneurysm. 'No point in assuming what went wrong,' 2IC nobly said. 'Let's see what the MRI tells us. You're very lucky, Mr Iannella!'

During the meeting, they advised me that the grinding sound in my ears was a condition called tinnitus, which is common in people who have worked with noisy machinery or have been subjected to loud noise for long periods at a time, like a musician. *Strange, that. I'm a musician.*

'But the noise is so loud.' I had a few questions, an opportunity to exercise my jaw muscles and turn thoughts into words. 'It's as loud as I can hear you speak,' my words came stumbling out. 'Will that go away?'

'We don't know.'

The examination was thorough, full of nasty discoveries. With some basic tests, they were able to determine that hearing in my right ear was gone. Kaput. Bad news comes in threes, as they say: 1) right eye staggering and stuttering, 2) the right side of my smile was droopy, and 3) right ear deafness. The opposites—*my body was predominately affected on the left, and my head on the right, weird.* It was another blow. *Sure, kick me while I'm down.*

'The hearing damage could possibly be related to the medication that was administered in Vietnam.' I didn't think I really needed to hear that last bit. 'It has side effects linked to hearing damage.'

As upsetting as that news first was, once I thought it through—rolled it around in my head again and again, then again—I came to the relieving conclusion that it wasn't so. One of the first telltale signs of my stroke had been the rumbling sound I heard in my ears even before I stepped off the bus at the tunnels in Vietnam, not to mention all the confusing sounds I'd heard before we reached Saigon in that rural medical clinic beside what I'd thought was a freeway or airport—*large trucks or planes rushing by.*

Coming to that understanding eased my mind. It made perfect sense to me. I didn't want to entertain the idea that my hearing damage that was causing me such great distress could have been avoided.

Relief.

The medically intriguing condition of my eye movement earned me the unofficial title as the hospital's 'Patient with Amazing Eyes'. It's not like I have eyes like Bette Davis, or old blue eyes himself Frank Sinatra, but more the subject of medical curiosity.

It generated a mass entourage of ophthalmologists, student doctors, inquisitive onlookers, anyone and everyone. They were endlessly probing, poking, pulling, squeezing until I realised it was all purely for the interest of research rather than my health. Though I was all for progress, the attention exhausted me. I soon refused being the subject matter of medical development and only allowed the Rowing Team to look over me.

The Patient with Amazing Eyes needed a nap.

SIX

# The Dungeon

With the amount of time I spent under daily soft interrogations by the Rowing Team—answering their questions, attempting to pronounce big medical words (and failing miserably), speaking to nurses and glorifying the minute-by-minute details of my demise to family and friends—I was making some improvements. 'Your speech is getting better,' my sister noted.

Suddenly, over the space of a few days, my vernacular was king of the hill. Sprinting ahead of all my other deficits, coming in lucky last. Going from bad to good, but definitely not losing.

Better speech, however, didn't exactly mean better chewing technique. My rubber-band lips were now tight enough to prevent chin dribble, but with slack-jaw psychosis, the mass-produced hospital cuisine—that, as far as I'm aware, hasn't yet received a Michelin Star—required running through a blender for my culinary delight.

A soft-serve diet, they called it.

The coordination of my shaky right hand played a pivotal role in decorating my bed sheets with mashed spaghetti. Forking food into my mouth had the fluidity of parallel parking a lorry. 'Hey, let me do it for you.' Occasionally, if one of my sisters was visiting during mealtime they'd lend a hand, feeding me like they once did when I was a bub. Gotta love big sisters!

Developing new skills doesn't take long. Discovering workarounds is human nature, in our DNA, evolutionary. I have some words for whoever designed those small square one-use plastic margarine containers. You know the ones—they have airtight sealed tops that require the aid of someone with the smallest hands on the planet to help you peel them off.

Those things need to go back to the drawing board and be redesigned to take into account those with one semi-functioning hand.

This is where the work-around comes into play—evolution. Like a bear ripping the head off a freshly caught river trout, I used my teeth to tear that top off. But removing the wrapper wasn't the frustrating part.

Trying to soften the concrete-like margarine in order to spread it across soft-as-marshmallow white bread without it looking like your dog just dug up your garden is!

Everything on my dinner tray was either sealed, screwed, glued, nailed, bolted, or welded shut. Drink containers, cutlery, napkins, salt, and pepper sachets, *everything*. Time was spent calculating mathematical equations on how the hell I was going to open things: using my teeth, my hands, a crowbar, a grenade, or calling in the army.

*So, this is what it'll be like living with a disability!*

The Rowing Team found that the latest MRI had failed to clearly show the degree of damage caused by my haemorrhage. *Do they even know what they're doing?!* I fumed silently. There was still substantial blood around the area that hadn't drained completely.

'We'll book you in with Radiology for an angiogram in a few days.'

I don't know if you have ever had an angiogram, or even know what one is. Well, I have two words to describe it: friggin' horrible!

As with all medical procedures, I had to fast for twelve hours prior. No blended breakfast, which was a breeze for me, as that's roughly about how long it took to rip open the sealed, screwed, glued, nailed, bolted, and welded shut food packaging.

There were eight helping hands assisting with transferring my *severed-string body* from one bed to another. Three nurses and the radiologist were there to collect me. He got to stretch his legs, soak up the daylight streaming in through the ward's massive unopenable windows as he ventured up from the hospital's dungeon basement where patients had their insides photographed, radiation zapping through their bodies.

A reenactment of my mummified routine was required as they slid me across the Bondi short board, known in medical terms as a transfer board—a piece of *four-foot-long, two-foot-wide plastic*—into the waiting transportation bed positioned beside.

Flashes of fluorescent light whizzed past. I lay motionless, mummified, blankly staring at the rolling ceiling. The radiologist, at the head of my bed, weaved me through hospital hallways, manoeuvring around corners, obstacles, trolleys, and morning breakfast cart. Glimpses of random conversations blurred by, muffled, as hospital staff stood idle, chatting, discussing all things medical.

*Ding,* the elevator bell sounded. Doors opened into the lift, then B was pressed on the numbers board and doors closed. Down we went into the hospital's dungeon.

It felt like a welder's workshop, a baker's kitchen, an underground car park. In a word, *unsettling.* I have a lingering visual image in my head of the room lit in blue, a visual image from when I could only understand things within a foot in front of me. It was far too much information for my lagging brain to process far too soon. I tried uselessly to wrap my head around it, decode it.

'Just lie still. Relax,' he said so leisurely, like I had a choice. 'It's going to take about an hour.' My anxiety was throttling—fight or flight started kicking in. I hadn't been told what an angiogram was, what they needed to do, or how. Flying from the seat of my pyjama pants, I was at the mercy of these *medical professionals,* in their hands. *Lie still, lie still.*

'I'm going to give you a local anaesthetic to numb the groin area.' All my attention was dead focused on what he was saying, words further muzzled through his blue surgical facemask. 'Just relax.'

The idea of the angiogram was to inject dye into my brain, then the X-ray machine would photograph my head. The dye that circulated through my brain's vascular system would be highlighted by the X-rays, showing the damaged area.

'I'm going to shave your groin, then make an incision. Keep still.' A diagonal two-centimetre cut was made across my skin, intentionally deep enough to slice open an artery called the aorta, the main vein that runs through our bodies and feeds blood to our heart and head.

This is the *friggin' horrible* bit: Through the incision, the radiologist inserted a small object they call the 'vessel'. Pushing it up my aorta from my groin to under my rib cage, beside my heart and onto the base of my skull around the neck region. Attached to the vessel was a thin tube line which delivered dye, pumping it into my brain.

'You're going to feel a warm sensation to the back of your head. Don't panic, it's just the dye doing its work.' *Fight or flight.*

I shut my eyes. *Let this thing be over, please!* The warm sensation circled around in my head, muscling its way in, crawling like a spider through my brain. Warm, creepy-crawly, disorienting.

I opened my eyes and wanted to vomit. *Suck it up.* Within my one-foot visual range, staring me right in the face, was the X-ray machine. I watched it dart around, pivoting back, forward, left, right, ensuring every angle of my head was photographed, X-rayed. *Radiation zapping through bodies.*

Upon completion, the X-ray machine pulled away to my side, retracting to its resting position. 'Take a moment to rest. The machine's finished X-raying.' I took a few deep breaths, trying to calm my throttling anxiety. Mounted to the wall adjacent to me was a row of LCD screens. Splashed across the screens were what appeared to be images of the inside of my head, a roadmap to my brain.

'Just keep still. I need to apply pressure for a few minutes to the incision so it closes up.' *Breathe.*

Venturing back up from the hospital's dungeon basement, welder's workshop, baker's kitchen, or underground car park, I heard a *ding*. The lift doors opened and someone started manoeuvring me out of the elevator and into my ward, weaving through hallways, dodging obstacles, the tea lady, the cleaner, the trolleys. The radiologist was again at the head of my bed, stretching his legs, pushing, pulling, yanking. Fluorescent light whizzed by; I did some blank staring. Nurses were idly chitchatting, discussing all things medical.

Back in my room, we entered into quietness, stillness. 'Try not to move for a few hours so the wound doesn't open up.' A bandage dressing covered my incision.

I was left alone to rest, take it all in. I added the footage to the silent movie in my head.

It was fairly early when the Rowing Team sailed on in to see me the following morning, shortly after breakfast. I must have been the first one off the rank for their daily routine visits.

They entered my room with an energy of disappointment, all six of them wearing blank faces. 'The angiogram results are inconclusive,' Head Doc sombrely said, the Coxswain. 'Blood still hasn't cleared for us to determine what happened.'

*They really don't know what they're doing!*

'Let's address it at a later stage.' Still no answers. 'We'll need to do the angiogram again.'

*Nooooooooooooo!*

'But for now, let's move on to rehabilitation.' His tone turned to optimism. 'The therapy team will drop in to see you over the next few days.'

*It was all I had thought I needed: my family by my side, finally. But not having answers to the how, why, and when of it all still left a gap, a hollowness.*

Before leaving, the Rowing Team waltzed through the same old dance routine: follow the finger, touch your nose, pinpricks, pushing, pulling, squeezing. I only scored a five with the panel of judges. My heart just wasn't in it; my mind was elsewhere, abandoned by the dance floor. Waiting, waiting, waiting.

I desperately wanted, needed, to hear some kind of explanation. A step-by-step plan, a map to recovery drawn on a large whiteboard with black marker using diagrams and pie charts indicating what would happen next, if I would be okay, how I would recover and if I would walk again.

The inconclusive angiogram was a puncture to my already deflated tyres, sucking the last bit of air out. I had built myself up, expecting to know and finally have some answers, a reason.

*Give me something to cling to.*

So, here it is in layman's terms, black and white: There was no one single answer. Nobody could say for sure; no one really knew. All the questions I asked were answered with *Possibly, Maybe, Could be*, or *We can't be certain*. Then, they would neatly conclude with this sweet bit of assurance: *The body has amazing healing ability!*

What it boiled down to was, scientists know more about our galaxy, thousands of light-years away, than the actual tool they used to imagine the possibility of such great discoveries—the human brain!

Through the course of the first three or four days in hospital, I had a steady flow of visitors. Family, friends and work colleagues all came to see me. 'How ya doing, mate?' It was all quite moving. It touched my heart to see them all, have their support, and know they cared. Loved.

Life moves quickly; we're all always too busy. Workloads, family commitments, raising children, renovating and so on—go, go, go. But then suddenly, unexpectedly, tragedy happens to someone you know, and you're faced with confronting your own mortality. Questioning, *What is life really all about?*

I lay in my hospital bed those days, tears streaming down my face while telling my closest friends, dearest family and nearest work mates the step-by-step details. The moments before, the rush to Saigon, the ICU, the rescue flight.

Openheartedly they listened, ears primed, faces shocked, teary-eyed. I felt their sincerity. It was beautiful.

'Hey, bud, I'm doing ok, feeling a bit better. I start rehabilitation tomorrow.'

The first assessment by the physio team was educational, truly 'thrown into the deep end' type of learning. They explained the process of rehabilitation, covering some of the techniques they'd be using to help me regain movement and strength—*diagrams and pie charts.*

'It's a slow and gradual process.' She stood close and spoke compassionately. 'It'll take time, slowly, bit by bit.' I felt a tiny flutter of hope. 'You know, the body has amazing healing abilities.' *So I've heard.* 'But first things first, we need to get an understanding of your strength. Let's do some tests.'

We ran through the dance floor favourite 'pinprick, pushing, pulling, squeezing' routine. Straight tens this time.

'Okay, we're going to get you out of bed.' My butterfly hope fluttered its wings. 'There'll be one of us on each of your sides, so don't worry you won't fall.' The wings started nervously flapping. 'We'll place your arms over our shoulders for support and then we'll stand you up.'

Together, they carefully manoeuvred me into an upright seated position on the bed's edge. Six helping hands this time.

Before I crumbled like a house of sticks—three little pigs, huffing and puffing—two of the physios promptly moved into a seated position either side of me, sardining me in.

They placed my arms across the back of their necks, shoulders wedged into my armpits. 'Okay, on the count of three we'll slowly stand.' I had a flashback of my enema—*rock, paper, scissors.*

'One, two, and three.' We were up. I was standing, propped up by two support bodies, sardined. My torso dangled like a bed sheet suspended on a clothesline, flapping in the wind.

'Good, good! Steady, hold still.' The floor below my unregistering bare feet felt like it was missing, hollow and empty. 'Slowly, slowly ... good. Let's try a step.' The room began spinning, turbulent. 'Don't worry, we've got you.' *Words spoken through a muzzle,* a rotating muzzle.

'Okay, left leg forward, lean and then right step. Good, good, you're doing really well.' I just wanted to get back into bed. 'Do you feel okay? Just a few more steps.' I begged silently for something to stop the room from spinning, to let me curl up into a ball and vanish.

To get the recovery rolling along, whilst angio #2 was on hold, awaiting further blood drainage, the physio advised I would be transferred into a rehabilitation ward, either there at Royal Melbourne or at Sunshine Hospital in the western suburbs.

'Sunshine Hospital ... really?'

If you're not familiar with the Melbourne suburb of Sunshine, let me inform you. The name doesn't describe the suburb, to say the least.

'Yes. Their rehabilitation ward is one of the best around!' She sounded convincing. 'They have a highly trained team'—upselling—'an impressive up-to-date gym'—closing the deal—'and their own hydrotherapy pool. They'll look after you!' Sold!

'You should be moved there within a few days.'

SEVEN

# Mamma Mia

Public perception debunked! Another casual ambulance chaffier ride—no siren required—across Melbourne's west and we were headed into the sunny suburb of Sunshine.

'Acute Rehabilitation Ward.' I only noticed the large sign above the entrance months later. I hadn't seen it the first time around, even though it was *blank* staring me in the face.

The paramedics pushed the gurney through the doors and into the ward.

'Which room is he in?' they asked the greeting nurse.

'Just through here.'

Blinding daylight streamed in through the floor-to-ceiling windows, its brightness bulldozing everything else in the room. My vision's aperture swiftly adjusted, closing, minimizing the entry of light.

Rehab was on the first floor, giving us a semi-panoramic view across Melbourne's western suburbs. 'Rooftops as far as the eye can see,' someone said. Not having to contend with inner-city suburban traffic made Sunshine Hospital certainly a more convenient option.

Once my vision stabilized and found *opaque* focus, I began familiarizing myself with my new surroundings. You know the drill: *light fitting, or air vent?* Considering I was only in the quad share room for a few days, for some reason—I don't know why—I can clearly remember the positioning of my bed, closest to the door on the right. Maybe my paranoia lingering.

*Wow, I'm not the only one.* As far as I could tell, it appeared my roommates, whom I assumed also had strokes, were all quite young. *So it doesn't only happen to old people.* Something I and many others believed—*'Stroke? But you're so young!' I often heard that at the beginning of my recovery. Even thought it myself.*

Debunked!

At that point, none of the doctors or nurses had elaborated on how or why someone has a stroke, who it could happen to, or at what age, and due to the inconclusive angiogram—*They really don't know what they're doing*—along with stubborn stale blood not yet ready to leave the crime scene, I was feeling a bit like a mushroom, left in the dark. So, when the paramedics rolled me into the light-bathed rehab room, once my vision balanced, I was quietly shocked by the youthful appearances of my roomies—*it's reported that even babies in utero have suffered from this awful disease.*

The nurse diligently settled me in, placed my belongings into the bedside drawer, entered information into my medical file, fluffed my pillows, and poured me water. No communication confusion. 'Press the call button whenever you need anything,' she said, making me feel right at home—*where everyone speaks English.*

I admirably watched her fuss around, doing what she could to welcome me to the fold and provide a sense of safety, security. *You'll be okay here. We'll look after you.* Though those words were never spoken, her actions were all I needed.

*This is it. This is where I'm going to be for a while.* A large part of me was keen to get started, get on with it, reclaim my life—*almost rubbing my hands together, thinking, 'Bring it on, I can do it.' It might take me a year or so, but then I'm done. Next challenge, please!* But the rest of me just wanted to disappear—to *curl up into a ball and vanish.*

'First, there'll be a physical assessment by each of the therapists,' advised the nurse, running through the list. 'You'll be seen by a physiotherapist, speech therapist, psychologist, stroke doctors, occupational therapist and a team of assistants.'

*Did she just say 'occupational therapist'?* was my first thought. *I just had my stroke, and they're already trying to get me back to work!*

'So, what's occupational therapy?'

'Occupational therapy focuses on your motor skills, like brushing your teeth, dressing yourself and holding a knife and fork, that sort of thing.'

*'Deep end' type of learning.*

'Rest up! Tomorrow will be a busy day.'

'The west is the best,' one of my work mates used to say. Relocation to Sunshine Hospital meant visitors were aplenty.

Friends often dropped in, distant family lavished me with chocolate, and work mates provided office gossip updates, told stupid jokes, and brought me lunch. 'Bud, I hope you like Big Macs.' Lukewarm and run through a blender, they still taste the same! A box of Krispy Kreme donuts, hand delivered with a smile and wrapped in best wishes, soft enough to eat without mashing it into baby food. There were cards, gifts and flowers sent. I even had an impromptu visit from the hospital chaplain, and she prayed for my speedy recovery.

*The incredible strengths of human kindness.*

Her approach was much slower, step by step. Probing, investigating, testing my strength, making mental notes, determining how to mend my broken body, my battered spirit.

'Are you feeling dizzy? Can you hear me okay?' Sincere and subtle, she had her own unique dance routine. One I instantly warmed to, desperately needed.

She perched me up on the edge of the bed, then promptly repositioned herself seated close behind me, in tandem, nestling me in between her legs. A secure hand braced my torso upright—*three little pigs, house of sticks*—holding me in position, preventing my body from crumbling.

'Is it okay if I remove your shirt so I can get a good feel across your back?' In my mind, I had already handed myself over, given her full permission to do whatever was required. My guard was completely down; I had no defences left. 'Yeah, sure.' Shaky and awkward, I thumbed the buttons, one-handed, through their holes on my flannel pyjama top. She wiggled it from my shoulders and laid it upon the bed.

'Excuse my cold hands.' I heard the sound of two palms shuffling together back and forth, trying to generate heat. The noise emulated what I heard in my head, between my ears—*a condition called tinnitus*.

Through my polar opposite sensations—heightened sensitivity and complete numbness—I felt her warm gentle hands rest at the base of my spine, pausing there for a moment. I felt her touching, feeling, administering contact Reiki, then slowly working their way across my entire back, energy transferring.

Fingers spread-eagled, almost in a basketball grip, her healing hands moved around to my rib cage. 'Just relax. Move with me.' She began to gently guide my upper body, twisting my torso on the ball of my spine. 'That's it, nice and slow.' The repetitive movements were minor, a few centimetres. Left side forward, right side back, right side forward, left side back, like she was trying to unhinge my torso from my lower half. 'Straighten your shoulders.' My disjointed body was like a *floppy mannequin, a severed-stringed puppet* as she manipulated me like Play-Doh, moulding me like clay, applying strategic physio techniques. I surrendered, intoxicated by the challenge, trying to breathe through the fog, the heaviness, the reality—*one-foot vision, rubber-band lips, cling-filmed face, Charlie Watts*.

'I'm going to sway you from side to side,' she said, cautiously changing course. Her suggestive instructions softly coaxed me from left to right, spine ball pivoting, teetering me on the edge of collapse, the parameters of my absent ability. She studied my core structure like she had X-ray vision, *making mental notes.*

It felt like we were doing nothing, just slow dancing from a seated position to an imaginary love song, swaying from side to side, buttock to buttock. 'Gentle, slow, easy … pause, hold … and back again.'

The physical assessment went for about forty minutes—thirty-nine minutes too long, in my opinion! Lots of questions were asked, many of which I had already answered a dozen times before with the Rowing Team in the Purana Files. By the end of the session my emotions rumbled like a volcano, boiling me into a poached egg, fragile on the inside. 'You better hurry and get me walking. I've got a marathon to run next week,' I said, trying to cover up my vulnerability with humour. But it wasn't funny. No one was laughing.

Standing at the threshold of rehabilitation, metaphorically, I was about to enter *the unknown, the darkness*—the recovery. With what vision I had, all I could see was the enormity of what lay ahead, the fear I had in my heart, the pain I felt across my body. The physio assessment uncovered the harsh realities, the dark truths, confronting me with the distance between where I was at and where I wanted to be.

'Tomorrow, I'll take you to have a look at the physio gym.' Kiwi, blonde, All Blacks. *Sincere and subtle.* 'With the other therapists we'll set you a schedule, a daily rehabilitation program.' Dark truths with a hint of hope. 'Once that's in place, we can start getting you better.' Smiling. 'First, we'll work at regaining your core strength, waking up those muscles that help you sit up, then slowly work on movement. It's going to take time, slowly, day by day.'

Walking wasn't mentioned; she didn't say if it were possible. Although tempted to ask, I refrained. The dark truths already revealed were enough one day; my poached egg self was still soft on the inside, fragile. *Maybe it's too early to tell anyway.* Patience, patient, patience.

'I know this is very emotional for you, but we need to push through.' She could sense I was trying to cap my volcano, keep the cork from popping, prevent my eggs from scrambling. 'We have to work hard and stay positive!' Sound advice. Honest, reliable, as solid as a rock—the Rock Goddess!

Next up to bat on the therapy assessment order was Long Arm OT, the occupational therapist—not there to hurriedly get me back to work!

From our very first meeting I sensed her openness, a softness and a calm about her. 'Are you okay? How are you feeling?' She asked like an old caring friend, her hand gently resting on my forearm. A gesture granting me a comfort to let my feelings flow, to allow my tears to fall as they may without fear of judgement.

It was like someone had turned the lights on, had pulled back the covers. She became my confidante, my soundboard, and my all-things medical adviser, answering many of those questions the Rowing Team had shrugged off with *Possibly, Maybe, Could be, or We can't be certain.*

Without hesitation, Long Arm gave me my first real hint of hope. A much-needed shot in the arm, an antibody full of possibilities—*something to cling to.* She provided me with documented examples of recoveries that other stroke survivors achieved … 'stroke survivor'. Wow—two powerful words, but they pack a mighty punch! I didn't think I had ever strung them together in a sentence, and I definitely never ever imagined I would be labelling myself with them.

*I'm a stroke survivor.*

'We'll start therapy tomorrow.' I liked her no-time-to-waste approach. 'We'll first begin by gaining an understanding on what you can feel. You know, like sensory and touch.'

Stroke had blown me out of the water, detonating beneath me, sending me hurtling into space. Listening to her speak began to gently return me back to Earth. A safe landing may still have been a long way off, but my parachute was now beginning to open.

'Then we'll test your strength, movement and function, focusing on hand-eye coordination and sensory stimulation.' The language was all so unfamiliar to me—not part of everyday conversation. 'We'll also work on feeling objects in your functioning hand, then passing the objects into your affected hand.' A foreign language, but I was understanding every single word; it was music to my one good ear. 'With your functioning hand, I'll get you to hold the object, paying close attention to how it feels, its shape, the edges, the temperature, its weight. Then, you lock those sensations into your memory.' I was like a sponge, taking it all in, sucking it up. 'When you pass the object into your affected hand, you also send the memory of how the sensations felt.'

It all sounded super sweet to me—fascinating, in fact. Every word she spoke continued to slow my fall from space. At lightspeed, I was learning the new language.

'This therapy technique is known as memory transferring. It's designed to reconnect communication between brain and limb!' I was keen to get started—*a much-needed shot in the arm, an antibody full of possibilities, something to cling to!*

'So, what was Vietnam like?' It was the first time I had gotten to reflect on the fun part of our holiday. *Oh, yeah, that's right ... we were on holiday.* The BS period.

That cruise across the Mekong River was truly amazing. A small group of eager travellers, open blue skies, the fierce yellow sun, an old rickety boat, caramel-coloured waters, rural farming villages. Getting to witness how they lived, watch how they worked. Just spectacular, brilliant.

The question about our holiday was a cunning ploy. The speech therapist's interrogation had a social angle to it, a devious plan. As I spoke, she stared at my lips, examining how I moved my jaw, listening to my tangled pronunciations. She kept me talking, asking questions and genuinely wanting answers. 'What was the food like?

How about the weather? Are the beaches nice?' Then she'd add her notes to the Purana Files.

'I've got this sandwich for you. I want you to take a bite so I can assess the way you chew.' Most of the Michelin Star-less food—the *soft serve*—I had eaten thus far didn't require much chewing. 'Do you like ham and cheese?' My taste buds weren't exactly in tip-top shape around that time, so whether the sandwich was ham and cheese or pickles and peanut butter, mashed, blended, pureed, it didn't really matter to me. It all tasted like tofu.

By the way—I have this theory as to how tofu was invented. My kids cringe when I mention the tofu theory. Deep in a Southern Chinese village, there was a farmer named Fu. He was trying to make his own blend of homegrown soy milk when his soybean mincing machine exploded, turning the beans into a rubbery solid formula.

Fu reached down to the floor. With a cupped palm, he scooped up the rubbery formula and thought, '哎呀, 那看起来像我脚趾之间发现的东西.' *Translation*: 'Gee, that looks like the stuff I find in between my toes.' Toe-Fu.

'Good, now chew.' Her face was about six inches from mine, well within my visual range. I could see her eyeliner, lipstick and mascara as she assessed my chewing rhythm. 'I'm going to put my fingers in your mouth. Keep chewing. Don't stop.' Two fingers, covered in blue latex gloves, moved into my mouth. 'Good, now swallow.' Her free hand at my throat, her fingers gripped my Adam's apple, feeling for the swallow. Interrogation.

'Well done, you're doing good. I think we can upgrade you from a mashed food diet to a diced soft serve meal.'

Don't get too excited—there's not a lot of difference between the two!

'Okay, I want you to practice blowing raspberries. Watch me. Put your lips together like this, then blow.' The function of my brain may have been compromised, but I didn't think I had needed a demonstration. 'Do them as much as you can. At least three times a day.'

Along with practising raspberry blowing, I had a neat set of facial exercises, lip pouting, eyebrow push-ups and jaw stretches to improve my right sided sagging smile.

'Are you blowing me a kiss?' asked the nurse early one morning.

'No, I'm doing my face exercises.' To add to the face flexing silliness, the speech therapist requested I also practise sounding out letters.

'P, P, P ... B, B, B ... O, O, O.' I'm sure I annoyed the guy in the bed next to me. He never said; stroke had stolen his ability to speak.

This ordeal was my first introduction to being in hospital. I never ever really got sick, had never had surgery, and had never even spent one single night in hospital before. I guess I was cashing in my medical chips all in one go.

I was amazed how everything is taken care of for you: meals, washing, laundry, even bedding. In the evenings, after visiting hours, there wasn't much to do other than watch the ceiling-mounted television. You could entertain yourself by flicking through channels, pressing buttons on the remote or summoning a nurse on call. Room service was at your fingertips—all that was missing was a minibar.

I reckon I developed stiff neck, lying there for hours staring at the TV. Thankfully it wasn't as confusing as watching Southeast Asian television—this time I wasn't the foreigner—but the picture was all fuzzy, like a flock of homing pigeons had defecated all over your aerial. And with the sound of Charlie Watts's drumming still ringing in my ears, the dialogue could have been in Vietnamese, for all I knew, because I struggled to grasp the storyline anyhow.

One evening I lay there blankly staring, neck stiffing, at the television. Not necessary watching anything, but more just looking at its shape, trying to follow the square outline of the TV unit, focusing on the picture, the colours, movement of characters on the screen. I may have been watching *Two and a Half Men* or something similar. I can't recall.

As I squinted my eyes, narrowing my vision at the TV and following its square box shape, I noticed that the wall of blur I was seeing had slightly changed. Whatever I was looking at seemed to now be trembling, ever so slightly but very rapidly. A tiny vibration, like the one you feel beneath your skin when nervous.

I began running my own tests, examinations. Looking across the room, I'd fix my vision on large objects: a chair, the wardrobe, a cabinet. Everything I looked at was taking shape. Still opaque, but there were lines, edges, squares, rectangles.

*It must be my trembling eyes that's causing the blurred vision,* I thought. *Why didn't the Rowing Team notice this ... and all those medical students who exhausted me with their examinations?! 'Follow my finger, how many fingers am I holding, pull my finger' ... what the hell!*

The next morning when I saw Long Arm, I wanted to show my confidante this wonky vision discovery I had made, the self-diagnosis. Hear my all-things-medical adviser's opinion, a lady I had just met but instantly trusted, *like an old caring friend.*

'That's fantastic!' Her energy was uplifting. 'I'll give you some eye exercises to do.'

My trembling irises, or rapid eye movement, is a condition called nystagmus, I was told later. Caused by a neurological problem, either present at birth or acquired after stroke, multiple sclerosis or trauma.

There is no cure.

Each doctor I saw through my recovery had their own particular dance routine. There were many alternatives, various styles. Some preferred the rumba; others, the waltz. The rehab ward doctor definitely favoured an improvised jazz solo from the 'no contact with patient' repertoire. One that looked like he was dancing to his very own rhythm, a beat that no one else could hear.

'So how are you feeling today, Mr. Iannella?' Almost every examination the Mechanic (the ward doctor) performed on me was executed from the foot of my bed. 'How's your hearing?'

Questions were asked where I'd have to reply with, 'What? Huh? I can't hear you, come closer.' The Mechanic examined me like I was an old Corolla, standing at the front of the car while I sat in the driver's seat, his head under the bonnet. *Yeah, mate, sounds like it's the fan belt. Gonna cost 'bout four hundred bucks. Can ya bring it in Chewsday?'*

When Tuesday came round, I wanted a full service, grease and oil change. *Get me up on a hoist and give me a good going over.*

'Doc, my hearing, it's so bad. The grinding noise in my head is driving me nuts.'

'Don't worry, you'll get used to it over time,' he said, wiping his hands with a dirty cloth.

'Is there anything you can do?'

'Perhaps try listening to music as a distraction. Use headphones—they'll help drown out the noise in your ears.'

While in Vietnam, the day before the line crossing, I bought a stack of CDs—remember, this was 2009; people still listened to CDs back then. Anyway, I picked them up from one of those dodgy street stall vendors scattered across the manic Ho Chi Minh City, the buzzing Saigon.

The guy sold everything you could ever imagine: Rolex watches, Ray-Ban sunglasses, Armani suits, Hugo Boss aftershave. If he didn't have it, he'd make a quick call on his Motorola flip phone fastened to his belt, and snap—'You wait here. I have friend.' Soon enough, one of his mates would come whizzing round the corner with what you're after, in any colour, size, variety, or version known to mankind.

This type of retail enterprise is the business model used for every two-dollar bargain variety shop in the Western world. It's the mothership.

So, I had my portable CD player, along with my enclosed over-ear old-school headphones, brought into hospital to give the Mechanic's suggestion a run around the block.

Now, the music I enjoy most is a little alternative, not so mainstream. The CDs I scored off that dodgy Motorola flip phone dude were from bands that I'd been listening to for years: Radiohead, Death Cab for Cutie, Gomez. Their music was very familiar to me, soundtracks to my life. But when I cupped those headphones over my ears and turned the volume up to eleven—*Spinal Tap* style—my brain did a backflip. It heard in reverse. Everything was warped, like a vinyl album left sitting on your car's dashboard on a blistering summer's day. *What the?* My ears weren't able to relay the music to my brain in the order it entered. *Desrever ... reversed.*

But I wasn't going to give up that easily. I couldn't abandon the one thing that always brought me joy, that made me smile: music! I figured I would try listening to songs that weren't so alternative, something with less distorted power chords and more soft synths. Something easier on the ears, gentler on the brain.

So, I began searching.

They've always been there. They'll never go away, guaranteed to make an appearance at every party for the rest of eternity. I remember watching them on our old black-and-white Rank Arena television. I fancied the brunette.

Mamma Mia.

EIGHT

# Bystander

The scent of disinfectant relentlessly lurked around the hospital, everything wiped dangerously clean, lifeless. Off-white walls, pastel furnishings, an empty vinyl armchair and a side drawer filled with an assortment of top-notch chocolate I was utterly uninspired to eat.

It was a stagnant marathon length. A short two weeks in rehab, a slow and thirsty fourteen-day pilgrimage across the barren desert to the Unpromised Land. With all my basic daily self-care needs resigned from my responsibility and reassigned to be facilitated by the nurses, my personal Grooming Guardians—and I do mean *all* responsibilities—I felt sidelined, watching from the bench. The first few days in rehab, they went as far as conducting the wiping component of that little task we all do while seated on a large porcelain bowl, with your pants down, in the smallest room of the house.

'Good morning, Mr Iannella, my name is Margaret. I'll be your nurse for the day.' I'd been relocated to another room, a twin share, with a window seat. 'It's time to get you up and ready for your shower.' I wasn't sure how she was going to manage that; most other attempts so far—*jackknifed, sardined*—had been nothing short of disastrous. 'I'm going to slide this harness under and around your body'—her eyes pointed down to the canvas potato-sack-like jumpsuit slung over her right arm—'then I'll loop it to the hoist above your head and airlift you off the bed and into the wheelchair.'

We both looked to the ceiling. She looked blank; I looked nervous. *Really?*

'It'll be right, don't worry. It's the safest way to get you out of bed.'

I wiggled my butt like I had ants in my pyjama pants, attempting to make myself weightless so she could easily slide the harness beneath me.

'I'll lean you forward so I can pull the harness over your shoulders.' The head end of my bed was raised, back supported by pillows. 'Can you fold your arms to your chest please?' Like I was executing a bungee jump, free-falling from a bridge. I placed my arms across my chest disjointedly. 'I'll just pull these loops in between your legs and attach them to the hoist ... okay, ready?' She pressed the Up button on the remote control. The hoist engaged, pulling the harness tight and enveloping me into a cocoon, swallowing me whole.

Ascend.

Wrapped like a burrito, I was suspended above my bed. 'Are you okay, Mr. Iannella?'

I was dangling from the ceiling, hanging in mid-air like an Italian salami my dad would tie to the rafters in his garage, curing, preserving. 'Yeah, I'm okay.' But really, I was just numb, empty, shocked with what my life had just become. *Oh my god ...*

Darkness. My elbows were tucked, fists clenched, wrists to chest, engulfed in a straitjacket type of harness, a human potato sack. 'Hold still,' she said, her voice attempting to remain calm, trying to ease my nerves.

The humming grind of the hoist, *mmmmhhhhh*, muted my emotions. It filled the room's silence, lifting me off the bed—*dangling salami*. A second of a pause. Stillness, only splinters of light piercing through the folds of the harness, then movement to my right, across. I was scrambling for any sense of perception, searching for a stable position, *numb, empty, shocked*. Another second's pause. 'I'm going to lower you into the wheelchair now, just hold still. We're nearly there.'

Descend.

He opted for the tried and tested manual transfer from bed to wheelchair single-handedly, solo. 'I'll lift you from the bed, *man*.' Shovel-sized hands, tall, Jamaican, pearly whites. If the Grooming Guardians were a football team, he'd be ruckman.

Like a hot knife through butter, he slid one arm beneath my back and the other under my thighs. With a single swift, effortless motion, he raised me off the mattress, cradling me into his tree-trunk arms and turning on his heels, then seamlessly lowering me into the wheelchair as if I were fragile fine china, precious. An acknowledging pat on my shoulder, a flash of his pearly whites.

He wheeled me into the dimly lit bathroom and straight into the shower recess. Butterflies fluttered in my stomach, anticipating the awkward moment ahead as he began to unbutton my hospital-grade flannelette pyjama shirt button by button, slowly, deliberately. He rolled the collar off my shoulders, peeling the shirt from my back and tossing it aside. Butterflies dancing, pearly whites.

Again, I attempted to make myself weightless as the Ruckman jiggled off my PJ bottoms and underwear between the wheelchair and my butt, tossing them onto the pile.

Removing the showerhead from its cradle, he pulled on the flick mixer tap. Water pulsed through the flexible hose and an open palm tested its temperature.

Caressing my skin, the warm water washed away my anxiety as it cascaded down my back, affectionately cleansing me. Clutching a soft sponge, his delicate shovel hand massaged fragrant soap all over my body. I smelt divine, like a bouquet of flowers. Gentle circular motions sent shivers up my spine, releasing nervous trapped butterflies, his pearly whites glistening in the dim windowless bathroom. We spoke no words, said not a thing. I remained silent, speechless—there's not a lot a bloke can say when he's naked and being sponged down by another bloke who's twice his size.

Soapsuds tumbled to the floor, billowed, dissolved and vanished into the drain. With a comforting heated towel, the Ruckman gently dried my warm wet body and dressed me in fresh clean pyjamas, threading my arms into the sleeves, folding the collar flat. Securing me button by button, slowly, pearly whites.

Positioning me in front of the mirror, he buttered my face with shaving cream and gave me a smooth, tight shave that most high street barbers would have envied. I was wheeled back into my room, clean, shiny and shaven. His tree-trunk arms swooped me out of the wheelchair. Our eyes met momentarily as he slipped me in between the fresh bed sheets. It was just beautiful, one-on-one, man-to-man, *uomo a uomo*.

Like the taming of a wild horse, the Grooming Guardians didn't waste any time breaking me into the daily hospital procedures. Wake, breakfast, medication, shower, bed made and rest.

With the morning out of the way, the afternoon began with bed, rest, lunch, rest, visitor, then more rest, and soon it was dinnertime. Then more rest, another few visitors and, you guessed it, rest. Followed by lights out and getting ready for bed for a good night's … rest.

Here's something I learnt very quickly: Do *not* mess with the nurse's schedule! Their finely oiled machine has been intuitively developed, artfully perfected through years and years of good old-fashioned elbow grease and cannot be altered; it can't be changed. You don't want to find a toenail in your tuna casserole or an old Band-Aid in your corn flakes? Just comply with the rules. *Smile and wave, boys, smile and wave.*

The precarious mission of showering was always an entertaining experience, a mixed bag of raw delights. Wiggle wiggle, jumpsuit, ascend, dangling salami, descend, button by button, soapsuds, a bouquet of flowers and all that in reverse, without the soapsuds, to get me back into bed. Then as I lay there in my birthday suit, void of any responsibility, they'd vigorously towel me down, ensuring that not one iota of wet skin was missed, as dry as a Salada biscuit. They got in and around my private bits without batting an eyelid—standard procedure for them, perturbing and awakening for me.

Dumbfounded.

My three young daughters would drop in for a visit after school with their mum, Charlotte and Molly still in uniform, their homework waiting, my heart breaking. Maddie, a few months shy of her first birthday and showing early signs of an adorably mischievous personality, would crawl all over my bed and touch everything she shouldn't.

My love for them throbbed with endearment while my spirit was staggered by the absence of being part of their daily routine. 'How was school today, hun?' I just wanted to be there, scrambling to find a car park close to the school, waiting for the bell to ring. To spot them from a distance as they headed to the gate, school bags casually slung over one shoulder, amidst the crossing lady, mums, dads, younger siblings, and prams ready to collect their little treasures and take them home for some family time.

Like a tornado ripping through a country town, picking up everything in its path and spitting it out wherever it may land, stroke doesn't discriminate. It scatters all those who stand too close to its whirlwind. It wasn't only me who had to make some major adjustments; my whole family was swept up, turned upside down, inside out and tossed to wherever they may land.

My fatherly duties had been forced to retreat for shelter through the storm: school runs, piano lessons, swimming, sports … all of it. And as I watched their mother single-handedly tow the heavy trailer load of parenting responsibilities, I could see her ropes were coming lose.

While she was predominately left to steer this sinking boat alone, most of the available life rafts were being used to keep me afloat, leaving her anchorless, lost at sea, aimlessly drifting. It was killing her. It was killing me. It was killing us. Like an *unmanageable weight,* an enormous amount of pressure was placed on our already ruptured relationship, our misfiring marriage. I felt helpless, while she felt abandoned, only advising me about her darkness many months later. 'Everything looked black. I just had no strength,' she shared, her voice trembling. 'I had nothing left to keep going; I couldn't do it anymore.' Her chin to her chest, eyes to the ground, tear-stained cheeks. 'There was a time I was on the shower floor crying ... I had no willpower to pick myself up.'

Like a hiker trekking the mountain ranges, carrying just enough supplies to sustain them for the treacherous journey. Step after step, day after day they battled through, running on empty. Supplies were scarce, enthusiasm was low, but they kept on putting one foot in front of the other. Tornado torn, aimlessly drifting.

*How's your brother doing?* My sisters braving a day at work, rearranging their busy lives to squeeze in a visit and trying to stay positive, supportive. 'He's doing okay,' they'd reply.

Between my brother, sisters and dad, a weekly visiting roster was coordinated. Monday: Sis one. Tuesday: Bro. Wednesday: Dad, and Thursday: Sis two. In no particular order other than who could get there, keep the morale up, pick up the pieces and mop up the tears.

'Dude, what are you wearing?' My bestie would sometimes pop in outside of visiting hours.

'I borrowed this white coat so security would think I'm a doctor.'

Work mates continued to visit, enlightening me with the shenanigans of home construction. 'Mate, you wouldn't believe what that numb-nuts of a brickie did.' This was a career I had stumbled into during my youthful years, my party days of travelling and living in London, working as a builder's labourer while trying to establish myself as a musician. And though employment in construction wasn't a consciously chosen path, I enjoyed the challenge.

After a half decade in London, slogging it out in a band in the evening and shovelling sand by day—'Ob-la-di, ob-la-da'. I returned home to Melbourne minus a music career but with a suitcase full of construction knowledge, and with some creative writing deployed to my CV, it jerried open the door into an unconsciously chosen career path. This led to a notable position in the domestic construction industry, all without me ever having to shovel Aussie sand.

It was the banter between work mates, being part of a team, I enjoyed most. 'Yeah, it's a little dry, mate. I would have taken it out of the oven sooner and maybe sprinkled brown sugar on top, so it caramelised.' Weekly meeting minutes about the cake one of the boys had baked for morning tea. 'Scott, it's your turn next week!'

A fortnight into this timeless recovery, I lay on my hospital bed beneath the matching pastel blankets, reminiscing, pondering, painfully discovering how all those things I had held so dearly in my life had now been hijacked. The dynamics were forever changed, as I was beginning to witness them continue without my involvement.

A bystander.

NINE

# Duke of Earl

'Over the coming weeks, I'll be conducting several varying tests which will include some basic thinking activities, a general questionnaire and eventually some more complex puzzles.'

The Duke of Earl embarked upon his honourable quest to tackle my battle-worn emotions by first declaring his defence strategy. 'And also lots of conversations and discussions about what you went through and how you're feeling.'

It was standard practice for all patients who suffered from a neurological disorder to be examined by the hospital psychologist. When the Duke first entered my room and introduced himself with an extended arm, anticipating a handshake, I didn't quite catch his name. It was different, uncommon, something that would have suited an old English gentleman of the monarchy.

The very first psych test I had with him was the questionnaire. Although he said the questions were of a general knowledge nature, they left me wishing I had paid more attention to my history teacher at school rather than sitting at the back of the class with who I had thought were all the cool kids. However, I gave it my best shot.

Question 1: Who was the Prime Minister of Great Britain during World War II?

Reply: Winston Churchill. *Too easy!*

Question 2: How many countries are in Europe?

I quickly began to name the countries out loud, counting them on my hand. 'Umm ... Italy, France, Spain, Germany, umm ... I thought you said it was general knowledge?'

It pretty much went downhill from there. I don't quite remember all the questions, but they were along the lines of 'Name all the oceans' and 'What's the capital of ... ?' All in all, I got a few correct, which satisfied the Duke.

'Well done.' He was grinning. Nodding.

His defence plan then progressed onto asking about my general health. I've always been a nonsmoker, and those days I only drank alcohol occasionally. If my room had a minibar, that 'occasionally' would have been right then and there, toasting the occasion with this charming English gentlemen. My guess? He's a G&T man. Otherwise, I kept relatively healthy, ate reasonably well and was physically active most days. Although the Duke never formerly announced it, I assumed all those factors excluded my lifestyle as a suspect.

'Is there any past history of stroke in your family?' Pen point pressed to his notepad, he awaited my reply. Neatly trimmed beard. Grey hair.

As I mentioned at the beginning of this book, my mother had had a minor stroke when she was alive. But her stroke was of a blood clot type, whereas mine was a haemorrhage. I didn't think the two were connected, but I mentioned it anyway.

While the Duke scribbled the information onto his notepad, like a surge of electricity, an epiphany, I remembered my aunty.

'Doc, my aunty suddenly passed away from a brain haemorrhage about fifteen years ago.' I said it with such conviction, as though I had decisively discovered the golden answer to 'why'. Mystery uncovered. Revelation revealed. *Someone call the Rowing Team—let them know that I've worked it out, and cancel that angiogram! It's a genetics thing!*

'Uh-huh,' said the Duke without lifting his head, scribbling in his notepad. Neatly trimmed beard. Monarchy.

Now that I've mentioned stroke types, this seems like as good a chance as any to elaborate a little more about the dark horse who's notorious for turning people's lives upside down.

We've all heard of stroke. But many of us, me included till now, actually don't know what a stroke really is—the specifics.

You may not be aware that there are *Different Strokes*.

'Whatcha talkin' 'bout, Willis?' That's right! Strokes come in two different types.

The first and the most common is an Ischemic stroke, the blood clot type. An Ischemic stroke occurs when a blood clot traps itself somewhere in a vein around the brain, preventing blood flow. As blood provides the oxygen required to revitalize our organs and cells, the clot deprives and starves cells of oxygen, leading to irreversible damage to the brain cells in the area of the stroke.

The second type of stroke, the one I had, is medically known as a haemorrhagic stroke, caused by a bleed or a burst vein, blood vessel, or artery in your brain, interrupting blood flow. The bleed suffocates and starves brain cells in the area of the burst, also causing irreversible damage.

I'll keep the dark horse's curriculum vitae brief. There's a PhD's worth of info that I'm not qualified to cover, but that gives you an idea of its skills and capabilities. For now, I'll just tell you one last thing: There is information stating that a section of the brain the size of a green pea dies every ten minutes when a stroke remains untreated.

Once the Duke finished gathering enough weaponry to potentially disarm the guerrilla warfare going on in between my ears, I had a few questions of my own. I was still grappling with the yet unanswered 'why it happened' question.

The evenings I spent alone, blankly staring at the ceiling-mounted TV. *Two and a Half Men* played fuzzily on the screen, not gripping me with its thrilling storylines of Charlie Harper's drunken debauchery and rampant womanizing. My mandatory inactivity gave me more than ample time to think everything over, and repeatedly—*I had many lengthy conversations with myself, a continuous internal monologue going till there was nothing worthwhile left to say.*

All the medical observations I'd had thus far indicated that my general health was in fairly good shape, *so why would someone have a stroke just out of the blue?* It just didn't make sense. *Could it happen again?*

The doctors were still holding their cards close to their chest, not giving much away. Now that I'd been in rehab for a few weeks, it felt like the emphasis on finding out 'why it happened' had shifted to 'fix what happened,' and though Long Arm instantly became my 'all-things-medical adviser,' she could only provide me with information trickled down by the poker-faced Mechanic. So, I attempted to pry some answers out of the Duke. Now that he had my back, in a moment of empathy, I figured, he may just lower his guard, relax the frontline.

'Doc, why did it happen? Could it have been from stress? My job's very stressful. Could that be the reason?'

But he didn't really have any answers. I was asking the wrong person, anyway; plus it was *still too early to tell*. I had to sit patiently, patient, patiently, and wait for my second angiogram before the Mechanic would play his hand. Bonnet down. Greasy smile.

So for now, it was business as usual, getting on with my rehabilitation. My roster was set and pinned to the wall beside my bed. It was a daily therapy schedule mixed with PT (physio), OT (occupational), ST (speech) and a weekly psych session. There were a few additional acronyms on my roster, ones I wasn't aware of and didn't know what they were for at the time: OTA (occupational therapy assistant) and WW (woodwork).

*Woodwork, cool ... maybe we'll build some funky furniture, or perhaps an outdoor entertainment area for the patients to enjoy. Oh, man, it's gonna be ace.*

'No, Antonio, we're gonna make a chopping board!'

Darkness. My elbows were tucked, fists clenched, wrists to chest. 'Are you okay up there?'

'Yeah, I'm fine.' The 'wiggle wiggle, jumpsuit, ascend, dangling salami, descend' voyage wasn't so adrenalilized with the Rock Goddess at the helm. She conducted the airlift with a cool demeanour, a collected calm. Plus, I had fast become a seasoned veteran—shower, airlift, toilet, airlift, bathroom, airlift—at being suspended from the rafters like my dad's homemade salami. Curing. Preserving.

The double doors were fastened open as she pushed my wheelchair through the threshold into the long and wide physio gym. 'Are you ready for your first physiotherapy session?'

I felt as eager as a teenager on his first date. I needed to get out of that pastel-coloured room, see a change of scenery, have everything wiped dangerously clean. It was a welcome relief to get up from the same position, lying flat on my back, prepared to ride the spinning room wave. Disinfectant lurking.

A dozen or so beds, the type commonly found in a masseuse's workshop, filled the spacious room, all with a hole cut out where you put your face while lying on your belly. Several beds were occupied by patients, physios reassembling severed-stringed bodies.

I did my now-standard room scan routine, familiarizing, attempting to iron out anxiety, and noticed a purpose-built set of steps standing solemn in the middle of the physio gym, towering across the room like a podium. Its appearance was intimidating, conflicting. The realism of my inability to climb those short three steps was difficult to conceive, another *dark truth* I wasn't yet ready to face.

'I'm going to slide you on your butt from the wheelchair and onto the bed.' In the Goddess's hands was a Bondi short board. *A one-foot-wide, two feet long piece of plastic, known in medical terms as a transfer board.* 'You just follow my instructions.'

She released the left bracket of the wheelchair arm and yanked it out of its sockets, then tucked the board beneath my left thigh, bridging the wheelchair to the physio bed. 'As I lean into you, I want you to place your chin on my shoulder.' Between Long Arm and the

Goddess, two ladies I had only just met, my life was in their hands. 'Then I'll brace my arms around you and slide you across to the bed.' My life in their hands, my heart in my throat. 'You just relax. Don't do anything—I'll do all the work! Don't worry, I won't let you fall.'

She stepped in close, bent into me and braced her arms around my upper torso. Chest to chest, collarbone to collarbone, my chin settled on her shoulder. 'Ready?'

We did the 'Harlem Shuffle' across the board, Bondi smooth. Then she effortlessly rolled me onto my back—*my life in her hands, my heart in my throat*—with my contribution at zilch, nada.

'Okay, take a moment to catch your breath. I have two student physiotherapists helping us for a few weeks. I hope that's okay with you?' After my previous bombardment at the hands of the medical students at the other hospital, poking and probing, trying to wring the first-handed perspective knowledge out of me, I was a little weary at first.

'Yeah, of course. That's fine ... hi.'

'Hi.' They seemed keen, friendly, open to absorb the Goddess's rich tapestry of experience. I kinda felt a little special, *cared for,* the centre of attention.

The three of them sat me upright on the edge of the therapy bed, with *my contribution at zilch, nada*. Acting as human airbags, the two students positioned themselves on either side of me, crouched beside the bed and tucked by my knees to act as fall barriers—*three little pigs, house of sticks, huffing and puffing.*

'Excuse my cold hands.' The Goddess got seated behind me, her shins compressed against the firm physio bed. She placed her hands on my back, *administering contact Reiki, energy transferring.* 'Okay, squeeze your left butt cheek and tighten those rib muscles.' I was slouched like a teenager in history class, compressed by the students. 'Can you straighten your spine?' Her fingers fanned around my rib cage—*spread-eagled, almost in a basketball grip*—her suggestive persuasion once again gently guiding me from side to side, buttocks to buttocks, my *spine ball pivoting* again and again and again.

'Good, good, slow and easy … move with me.' It still felt like we were doing nothing, just *slow dancing to an imaginary love song*. My legs hung over the bed's edge, bare feet resting on the imperceptible floor, while the human airbags stayed at my knees, fall barriers by my sides.

There I sat, totally dependent on these three people guardrailing me from falling, scaffolding my house of sticks. The first two or three physio sessions continued to uncover, roots and all, the *harsh realities, dark truths*. Myself, me, and I were gone—no longer there, no longer here. The distance between who I was and who I had become in a blink of an eye stretched far beyond my reach, unattainable. My faith was totally invested in Long Arm and the Goddess to close that gap, returning me to myself.

Like a thief cracking a safe, fixed and focused, the Goddess's concentration was unwithering. 'We need to awaken those deep abdominal muscles.' I don't think I've ever trusted anyone in my entire life more than I trusted her right there, right then, right at that moment. 'Head straight, chin up.' Like a Russian Olympic gymnast coach she guided me through it, deliberate, direct, disciplined.

This is where therapy had to begin: at the very bare-bones fundamental basics. Everything hinged on rebuilding a deep core strength and solid muscle foundation. Through each and every physio session, the Goddess would overemphasise their importance. 'Squeeze your butt, straighten your spine, tighten your rib muscles,' she'd repeat.

I had no idea how the process worked. I'd never seen a physiotherapist do their thing before, mending broken bodies—had *never been in hospital or had surgery*. The miles and miles between where I was at and where I wanted to be extended so far that I just couldn't work out how we were going to get there, to finally arrive home. In my wishful-thinking mind, my naïve brain, I hoped, prayed and desperately wished for it to be a quick and painless recovery, one that would reward me with rapid results. Within days, just a few physio sessions, and then BANG—I'd be up and walking!

But the Rock Goddess had other ideas. She knew better; she didn't rely on wishful thinking to get me back, to *return me to myself*. She said it how it was, *subtle and sincere* but honest, reliable, as solid as a rock. *'It's going to take time, slowly, day by day!'*

Although my first physio session wasn't exactly filled with an aerobic workout—*slow dancing to an imaginary love song*—my energy levels were depleted, drained like a mobile phone battery worn from a day's use without a charge. Exhausted beyond any human standard I had ever experienced through my BS life, the fatigue triggered an uncontrollable tremble in my left knee and wrist. Twitching like chattering teeth, an exaggerated case of the DTs. Once it got started, the damn thing wouldn't stop. My limbs had a mind of their own, the same mind as during the diaper explosion. It became a common phenomenon through most of the physio sessions; it happened every time and made me feel *yuck*, hammering home the state of my condition.

'It's the muscle not switching off.' The Goddess would apply pressure to my nerve endings, trying to persuade my 'mind of its own' to stop thinking for itself.

Occasionally, when being pushed through the physio gymnasium, I'd catch a glimpse of myself in the mirrors that lined one of the walls. A hazy outline reflected back, fuzzy, *defecated aerial*. An unnerving image, an uncomfortable sight. My once joyous self, full of life, agility, flexibility and health, replaced by a frail, fragile, rigid broken body. A man in a wheelchair.

I had to look away.

To relieve my DTs from the obnoxious chattering, I was allocated a break in between therapy sessions. An extended smoko to recover from the fatigue, giving me a chance to recharge my 'drained in a flash' battery.

Then it was back to the pastel-coloured room that just had a deep clean while I was gone—*disinfectant dangerously lurking*—through the airlift voyage on a one-way ticket. *Wiggle wiggle, jumpsuit, ascend, dangling salami, descend.* Then I'd have some downtime to extinguish the beyond-human standards of fatigue that characterised AS life.

Once the fire was out, it was back through the airlift voyage on a return ticket and into the gym for another round.

Stroke and fatigue are brothers in arms, thick as thieves. They stick together like honey and the bee, a united combo that zapped the energy out of me faster than Usain Bolt's hundred-metre dash.

It may have been my confidante or the Goddess who fed my need-to-know curiosity—it sure wasn't the poker-faced Mechanic—but the storage component of my damaged brain was able to retain the fatigue and stroke 'thickest of thieves, Dumb and Dumber' information in order for me to write this next section without researching whether it's correct or not. So, suffice to say there's a good chance I've ballsed it up.

In any case, here's what I remember: Muscle fibres are wrapped with cells that draw oxygen from blood, revitalising the muscle. With the lack of communication between brain and muscle caused by a stroke, the cells don't respond as required. Muscle fibres are then starved of oxygen and nutrients, subsequently leading to muscle fatigue.

I was concerned when Long Arm attempted the Harlem Shuffle with me. The dance across the board from wheelchair to physio bed required a considerable amount of muscle, and though she was a few months pregnant, she orchestrated the shift with incredible ease.

Bondi smooth.

'Careful, you're pregnant. Don't want you to hurt yourself.'

'I'll be okay. I've done this a thousand times before, you know.'

Raised to a forty-five-degree angle, I lay semi-upright on the physio bed. Long Arm was seated beside me, legs crossed and a clipboard nestled on her lap.

'What do you want to achieve by the end of your rehabilitation?' The question rolled off her lips without hesitation, like she had said it 'a thousand times before.'

I was taken aback, thrown off; it caught me off guard. As far as I was aware, I would be making a full recovery back to normal, and quickly—in a few days, I hoped.

I paused for a moment.

'Ha ... what do you mean? What do I want to *achieve*?' It felt like a trick question.

'We need to make a list of things that you would like to regain.' But judging from her face, she was dead serious. 'Like tying your shoelaces, buttoning your shirt, and so on, so that we can focus on those tasks.'

I wasn't quite sure how to respond. I needed to digest it for a second. The idea of not making a full recovery was one I hadn't yet entertained. The finer details of buttoning a shirt or tying my shoelaces were outside of my scope of consideration at that point.

'I'd like to walk, dress myself, hold my kids in my arms, drive and play the guitar again ... do normal things.'

'Are you a musician? Let's get someone to bring your guitar in. We can incorporate it into your therapy.'

That made me smile—wonkily, sunken downwards at one end (the right end)—but it was still a smile, nonetheless. *Great idea— the woman's a genius!* I could see the benefits. It made complete sense; combining the physical activity of playing a guitar and the love I have for music would surely result in a positive outcome.

*Someone go get my guitar. I've got a gig.*

'Let's get started.' Long Arm repositioned my bed so I was lying flat, down from the upright position. 'We'll work on sensory stimulation. I'm gonna place some hot and cold packs across your body, switching from one to the other, and I want you to tell me which is which.' She spoke in that medical language—*not part of everyday conversation*—a language I was becoming fluent in. *Sensory, stimulation, core strength, muscle memory.* Fluent in understanding, but not quite fluent in pronouncing.

'S ... s ... sen ... sss ... ooorrr ... r ... y ... y.'

It appeared that all the therapies I required—PT, OT, SP, OTA and WW—had to begin at 'bare-bones fundamental basics'—square one. I hadn't forgotten how to do those basic tasks like shirt buttoning, lace tying. My brain knew the steps required, understood how to do it. What I had to learn now was a new method, a different approach to retrain my old functions.

'Is that hot or cold?' She first started at my extreme left. Placing the packs in varying positions on my ribs, arm, thigh, hip and belly, she alternated between hot and cold.

'I don't know ... can't really feel it.' Then she moved from one side of my body to the other.

'How about now?'

'Hot, cold ... nothing ... warm, hot ... not sure ... cold ... ummm ...' In short, Melbourne weather. The sensations ranged from complete blankness to a feathery touch, a distant echo. There was a clear separation from my numb left side to a responsive right. A line could have been drawn right down the middle of my body, dividing it like the state of Western Australia and the rest of the country.

'Close your eyes. I'm going to poke you with this object, and you tell me where you can feel it.' We did the Hokey Pokey for a little while, frequently crossing the Nullarbor, stopping at random locations. I felt the changing of seasons: a heavy rain poke, a light-as-a-feather shower, a faint drizzle, nothing, something, something, then nothing, all weather conditions.

'Well done! Let's try some movement exercises.' All those crazy varying sensations flipped me out. I just didn't know my own body anymore, further exposing, *roots and all,* the gap between who I was and who I had become *in a blink of an eye.*

'I want you to raise your affected arm and reach for the ceiling.' As if I were an amateur ballerina learning *Swan Lake*, she slowly guided me through the movement. 'Steady, steady ... straighten your elbow and hold.' My arm extended upwards, the furthest it had stretched in weeks. Pointing to the ceiling, reaching for the stars, I was wobbly and shaky, like an old drunk longing for their first morning drink.

Sobering.

Later that evening, I was tucked into bed. PJs on, TV remote, call button, *Two and a Half Men* playing. Interrupting the monotony, a young woman politely strolled into my room.

'Hi, how are you? I heard what happened to you and wanted to tell you about my brother,' she began, her voice fragile. 'He's in the next room and had a stroke just like you.' I could feel my tears pending, building, ready to fall. 'It happened a few months ago. He's getting better, slowly, and soon he will walk again.' *The tears released. Falling. Flooding.*

She held my hand. 'Don't worry—you're going to walk again. You're going to walk out of here with my brother. We'll all walk together.'

TEN

# The Dungeon – Part Two

It was worth peeving off my roomie—those annoying morning vocal exercises got my talking fitness close to match ready. Everyone was commenting on my improving ability to speak.

'You're sounding much clearer, man! Less slurring,' my bestie commented, in for another after-hours visit.

'Dude, is that a nurse's dress you're wearing?'

'Yeah, I even shaved my legs!'

It was best to tackle big muscly words, punch them into shape with a slower approach, consciously pause for a second and take a breath. Then, I'd stage my rubbery lips as if I were about to recite *Macbeth* to prevent murdering the monologue. An eager delivery would often result in a mouthful of syllables all wrestling to become king. Lengthy words lingered in my head for too long, transfer suspended till my brain arranged the sequence of pronunciation, push-started a stumbling sentence and nudged forward the stalling speech.

As the days rolled on—*across the barren desert*—my time was occupied with acrobatic vocal gymnastics, blowing raspberries at the Mechanic, making pouting kisses for the Grooming Guardians and crazy man grins for the tea lady. An alliance with the crown of thorns, that had my head in a vice, had begun to form, an immunity against the feasting bull ants—*face taunt like cling film stretched over leftovers.*

Speech became the recovery darling, my rehabilitation's shining star, growing from stroke to strength. The little diamond was an inspiration for all my other deficits, who watched in awe, proud of their compadre, hopefully putting a rocket up their ... to do the same. Accelerate—*a quick and painless recovery.*

Like a firecracker, the fuse was lit. Improving speech ignited my confidence—*slack-jaw psychosis,* successful diagnosis. They couldn't shut me up. I was making up for lost time, asking about everything. 'Why? How? When?'

*Eyeliner, lipstick, mascara, blue latex gloves.* The speech therapist wasn't winging it—*two fingers, entering my mouth*—her cunning ploy, her devious plan, had a strategy. Soft interrogations had me waffling on like a POW revealing top-secret information.

Spitting P's, bumbling B's, rounding O's—as foolish as it may have sounded, and as silly as it made me feel, it was working.

'Insanity is doing the same thing over and over and expecting a different result.' —A. Einstein. Not this time, Albert.

I was stuck in first-gear therapy for a few weeks, square one, covering the bare-bones fundamental basics. The Rock Goddess was seated in her regular position, tandem, continuing to mould me like Play-Doh day in day out, manipulating, shaping, pivoting, twisting, turning.

Her master puppet hands controlling my *severed-stringed body*. 'Tighten those rib muscles. Straighten your spine.' She swayed me from side to side, buttock to buttock, again and again and again. 'We need to awaken those deep muscles.' Always *over-emphasising* 'it's the foundation of all movement,' giving me a physiology crash course. 'Without it you won't be able to sit, stand, walk or extend your arms!'

I couldn't see her seated behind me. She was always so quiet, deliberate, *unwithering*. I imagined her ear pressed up against my back, *like a thief cracking a safe*. Her movements were measured, precise, calculated, twisting me an inch one way, turning me an inch another. A long run-less bout of cricket innings, student physios fielding in slips—*human airbags, fall barriers.*

With frequent trips back and forth across the Nullarbor, my divided states, we went east to west, west to east, clocking up kilometres and stopping in all locations. OT sessions with Long Arm were persistent, *day in day out.* 'Hot, cold … nothing … warm, ummm …,' then switching to the Hokey Pokey. 'Can you feel this? Can you feel that?'

We progressed onto some simple Simon Says exercises, usually wrist flexing and finger bending. I often sat tucked beneath a school-sized desk, my torso supported by the wheelchair. Long Arm opposite me, we sat face-to-face. 'I want you to bend each finger forward.' My hand was a lump of limb, throbbing from the tiny jackhammers. 'Only move one finger at a time. Try to keep the others straight.' the concentration was consuming, depleting. 'Tighten those rib muscles. Straighten your spine.' My capacity to do two things at the same time, like sit up straight and bend my fingers, had been all but erased.

Scattered across the meter-wide school desk, laid out before me was an assortment of objects. A spoon, a knife, a paper cup, a ball, a block. Tools to retrain my brain.

'Pick up the spoon with your good hand. Hold it for a minute and memorize how it feels.' The concept of the memory transfer exercises felt like a Rubik's Cube, puzzling. 'Now, close your eyes and pass the spoon along with the memory of how it felt into your other hand.'

My lump of limb seemed illiterate, unable to read messages, create shapes or form a frozen claw hand. Commands for movement were muddled; it wasn't clear which finger did what, what finger did which. The cup was crushed in my hand, the spoon clattered to the floor, the ball went bouncing away.

This stagnant marathon, *across the barren desert to the Unpromised Land,* had only just began. My stamina was pushed to its compromised limits through every single waking moment of each and every day. All activities became energy vampires: the airlift, showers, physio, talking, eating, OT, SP ... all of it.

'Tighten those rib muscles. Straighten your spine.' I sat *slouched like a teenager in history class,* struggling to comprehend.

Bang on cue, like clockwork, bright and early—a *finally oiled machine, artfully perfected*—my Guardian raised the blinds, morning light spilling into the room.

I cast my eyes out through the spotless window, squinting to reduce the flood of light, and saw the hospital car park below—*rooftops as far as the eye can see.* Mindlessly gazing, *blankly staring,* I searched for any activity that resembled life, normality.

I now had a few weeks of what seemed like progress-less eyeball gymnastics under my belt. A morning ritual followed by spitting P's, B's and O's. Still not a word of complaint from my roomie, stroke not yet ready to hand his voice back.

But this particular morning, it wasn't such a stagnant start to the day. There was change on the visual horizon—a clarity on the looking front.

I began to zero in my focus on a few of the cars. A red sedan, a blue wagon, a silver four-wheel drive. I couldn't believe it, but there they were—a sea of vehicles neatly parked between white lines, side by side, left to wait for their owners to return. I could see details, shape, size, colour. People walking, crossing the road, looking left, right, then left again. Morning faces, a grey jacket, a black skirt, black shoes, a briefcase. *Vision!*

I turned on the telly, flicked through the channels. I stopped on a morning show and watched, clear and sharp, a way-too-perky-for-that-time-of-the-morning presenter, demonstrating how his titanium steak knives could easily cut through a leather shoe and how, if I called now, I'd get a second set free.

Bursting with excitement, a toddler on a red cordial rush, I thought, *I can see, I can see!* I wanted to shout it out across the sleepy-eyed ward, throw fist pumps into the air, slap someone a high-five, dance, kiss someone—so I kissed the nurse. I'm sure he would have preferred a handshake, but I was too happy to contain my joy.

I really did have ants in my pyjama pants waiting for Long Arm to get into work. I was itching to tell my confidante, to see the expression on her face.

*Someone order those steak knives, get the second set free! Let's have a party. I'm coming back, baby!*

Well, that joy was short-lived.

A few days later, Long Arm noticed my right eyeball beginning to migrate towards my nose, left of centre. I wasn't aware it was happening; it hadn't affected my vision enough for me to tell.

In that very short visual grace period, the frequency of my trembling irises—*nystagmus, involuntary rapid eye movement*—appeared to have slowed a little, beating at a heart rate pace instead, allowing my eyes enough time to capture sight and relay the footage onto my lagging brain.

From the inside looking out, I had sharper focus, giving my confidence an extra boost. I could see Long Arm's smiling face, watch the Goddess for her animated instructions, see the Guardians fussing around. I was better understanding my surroundings, the environment. I no longer felt the need to blankly stare at the ceiling anymore, and the pastel-coloured scheme of my room appeared brighter, richer. Objects that I had previously thought were light fittings turned out to actually be fire sprinklers.

Those simple realisations, determining objects, were personal rewards, gratifications, private pats on the back. It was a tiny step forward, providing me with a sense of warmer security. 'The body has amazing healing abilities'—the Rowing Team's catchphrase appeared to be ringing true.

The visual processing time lapse, with my *lagging brain,* had gladly improved. But as my right eye continued to crawl its way towards my nose, I began to see double of everything. Two Long Arms, two Goddesses, two Guardians and two Mechanics.

It further impacted my natural judgement of distance and space. The range of things I could see and understand had extended well beyond twelve inches, but now the pictures my eyes sent on to my brain were floating like helium balloons tied to a letter box at a garage sale. Confusing.

Long Arm pushed me into the bathroom and positioned my wheelchair in front of the mirror so I could see for myself. And sure enough, there I was, me looking back at me, cockeyed!

Over the following few days, the migration continued. My eyeball ventured its way, millimetre by millimetre, minute by minute, moving closer and closer towards my nose until it could move no more.

Continuing to dampen this momentous occasion, rubbing salt into the cockeyed wound, a series of bedside vision examinations were conducted by the Mechanic. A grease and oil change times two. 'Keep your head still and follow my moving finger with your eyes.' Bonnet up. Two greasy smiles.

From left to right, my wonky eyes began following his pointing finger. Both eyeballs scanned across, fixated on the target, tracking it in unison and departing together as a pair, a couple of eyeballs working as a team.

Then, along their follow-the-finger journey, as they both began to pass the centre of their eye sockets, my right eye decided to break the lifelong unison partnership. It wanted to go solo and do its own thing, free-spirited, stopping halfway in the centre. While my left eye obediently did what it was told, continuing to follow the Mechanic's moving finger and going on its merry lonesome way till it arrived at its destination, all the way over to the far-right corner. And once I looked straight ahead again, attempting to reunite my eyeballs, unify them as a team, my right eyeball resisted. It wanted to stay free-spirited, individual, an SLR—a single-lens reflex, returning back to its corner like a heavyweight boxer after the bell rings.

The 'one plus one equals two' vision meant my sights settings were in split-screen mode, left and right. I felt the same confusion as trying to watch Vietnamese ICU television—*Was it the foreign language? Well, the local language; I was the foreigner.* My brain's visual centre needed to decide which of the split screens to watch, which to follow. *Weird!*

This is where things got interesting.

With my newfound sight, though severely cockeyed and seeing everything as doubles—four hands, four feet, two drink cups—I now had enough visual ability to focus on a page of text to read.

By closing my free-spirited right eye, like a very long wink, it eliminated the eligible overlapping of text. The scrambled sentences, words and letters suddenly realigned, returning my sight to SLR status. Mono.

It was the same eye I'd had trouble closing while in ICU, the one the nurses had taped shut. I'm no doctor, but my guess is it was all related!

Now that my vision was well enough to read, cockeyed and all, Long Arm gave me an information booklet about stroke that kept me entertained for hours. I read it cover to cover, page after page, twice, in mono.

*After coronary heart disease, stroke is one of the largest causes of death in Australia and is a leading cause of disability. About 88% of stroke survivors are left with life-long disabilities. Stroke kills more women than breast cancer and more men than prostate cancer.*

Who would have known?

*Close to 20% of strokes occur to people under the age of fifty-five.* Another public-perception-debunking fact.

But the statistic that rattled me like a maraca was this: *One in five people having a first-ever stroke will die within the first month, and one in three die within the first year.*

Maybe it wasn't such a good idea giving me that information booklet!

'Will that happen to me? Will I die within a year?'

'You're not gonna die!' Even though I knew Long Arm couldn't make any promises, hearing it from someone I trusted enabled me to sidestep a tumbling avalanche rolling it around in my head. Plus, she added what was to become my favourite bit of advice: 'The body has amazing healing abilities!' *Yeah, so I've heard.*

The stroke information booklet only half satisfied my curiosity. I needed to know more. I didn't just want statistics; I wanted further details about where my stroke had occurred and why had it caused so much damage. I knew it was in my brainstem, but why had it almost killed me? Why couldn't I walk, talk, hear or see properly?

I reckon this was around the time I began to rub the Mechanic the wrong way.

Upon his next routine examination, I had questions that I needed answered. I wanted him to explain to me, in simple and easy-to-understand words, step-by-step, exactly how the hell the brain worked—well, 'exactly' or thereabouts. I had gathered enough information from the booklet to at least grasp some basic knowledge of its general function, but I wanted a professional to explain further—a doctor to clarify!

While he stood in his standard jazz solo-esque improvised dance routine position at the foot of my bed, he had his bonnet down, poker faced times two. Reluctant to hand out information, he was still holding his cards close to his chest. He vaguely answered my questions, only covering the need-to-know basics—*'Yeah, it could be the fan belt'*—then making a dash for the door as if stroke were contagious.

So, my interest was now only three-quarters satisfied, left salami dangling from the rafters of curiosity. During the 'I still read biology books about the brain ... hoping the flashing sign above my head broadcasting "MAN WITH DISABILITY" fades' period, and for the purpose of this book, I decided to research it myself.

This is what I discovered.

The brain, that wrinkly walnut-looking thing lurking inside our skulls, is known as the cerebrum. The cerebrum is divided down the middle into hemispheres, the left and the right. Each hemisphere has four identical parts called lobes: the frontal, temporal, parietal and occipital lobes. With one of these lobes on each side, this makes eight lobes total. Each pair of lobes has a specific function.

Memory, speech and reasoning are controlled by the frontal lobes. It contains our language centre, providing us with the ability to read, write and speak. The frontal lobes also allow us to think, reason and make decisions. It's the platform for our intelligence, making each of us uniquely individual.

The duty of the temporal lobes covers hearing, taste and smell. Our noses are directly linked to the temporal lobe, and the information we gain from taste and smell is processed here.

The occipital lobes are responsible for sight and visual processing. Information collected by our eyes is transferred along the optic nerve to the occipital lobe. Our eyes are like a camera—they record the information and send it to our brain for processing. In fact, we don't see with our eyes; we see with our brain.

Touch, feel and sensory processing are handled by the parietal lobes. Most of the information that comes from our senses, such as taste, sound and smell, are processed here so our motor skills can be coordinated. The parietal lobe gathers all the information and combines it into one complete package.

The eight lobes are all intricately wired with strands of tiny nerve cells. Information transmitters, known as neurons, crisscross and communicate with one another. They transmit the information along its communication pathways down into the brainstem and into the body, enabling us to function as we do.

The communication pathways are all compressed together and jammed into the space of the brainstem, which is about twelve millimetres in diameter, roughly the width of your little finger.

I have indicated in the diagram below where my brain haemorrhage occurred. The bleed I had in that tightly spaced area effectively suffocated and drowned my nervous system, disabling communication from my brain to my body and damaging vital brain cells.

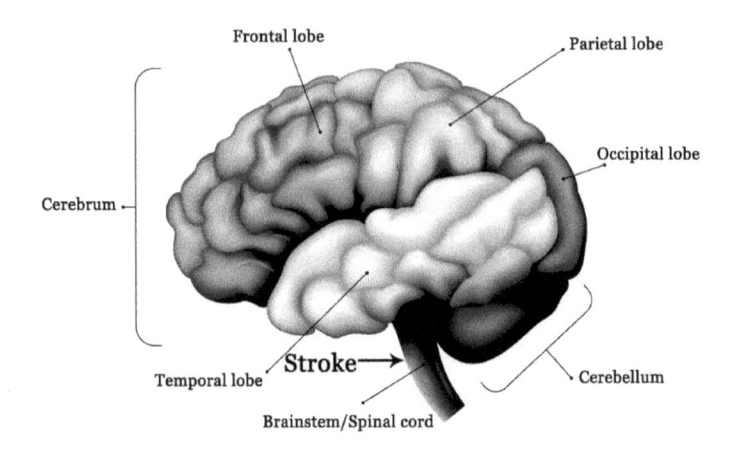

*Frontal lobe, Parietal lobe, Occipital lobe, Cerebrum, Temporal lobe, Stroke →, Cerebellum, Brainstem/Spinal cord*

The brainstem is also responsible for keeping the things we don't think about working, like our heart, kidneys and even breathing. We could survive without the rest of the brain, but we cannot survive without the brainstem.

'If you had the same-sized haemorrhage in another location of the brain, you may have only had a headache for a few days,' mentioned one of the doctors.

Now we know why it caused so much damage. The biggest question left was: Why did it happen?

My angiogram was scheduled for a few days' time.

The procedure room didn't look like a welder's workshop, nor did it feel like a baker's kitchen or an underground car park. It was bright, clean and sterile, glimmering with artificial light showering down from the ceiling. Modern medical equipment sat nearby, ready and waiting to investigate my insides. LCDs were pinned to the wall, reporting their findings.

I was placed beneath the machines, anticipating. 'Lie still. We're going to give you an injection to numb the groin area,' said a young doctor in surgical blues. 'Just relax.'

The spike of the needle pierced through my skin. My groin was instantly numbed, then shaved with a disposable razor. One use, discarded and tossed in the dust bin.

Like a dull nick on a barbwire fence, a paper cut, the surgical knife sliced open an entry point into my internals. Local anaesthetic blocked the pain.

The doctor began to push the vessel up my aorta—*the main vein that runs through our bodies and feeds blood to our heart and head*. Like a masseuse massaging out a nerve knot, I could feel the pressing of his knuckles digging into my skin as he pushed and pushed, threading the dye-delivering object higher and higher, deeper and deeper. Through my abdomen, up under my rib cage, beside my heart.

The knuckle digging stopped when the vessel arrived at its destination at the base of my neck. There was a long pause. 'You're going to feel a warm sensation in your neck region' came the scripted warning, I knew what was coming—*the friggin' horrible bit. Hold on.*

The warm, intoxicating dye flooded my brain like a tsunami—*muscling its way in, crawling like a spider*—as I tumbled through its dizzying current, trying to grab hold of stillness till the force subsided.

Hovering above my face like a satellite Google mapping the globe, the X-ray machine repeatedly darted around, snapshotting my head—*radiation zapping through bodies*—then resigned, parking itself to my side upon completion.

Eyes wide open, harvesting the moment, I tried grounding myself—*fight or flight*. The LCD screens pinned to the wall on my left again displayed the roadmap of my brain, freeways, highways, streets and tiny lanes zigzagging all over the place.

The radiologist wheeled my bed out into the waiting area, then applied pressure to the incision to close the wound. He looked down at me and said:

'I know you. You're that bloke who had his stroke in Vietnam!'

ELEVEN
# BS Period

Whenever I used to hear the name 'Vietnam,' like a landmine of dormant year-nine social studies knowledge, the first thought that detonated in my mind was the war.

Thirty-five years had passed since Saigon fell to the communists, and decades after a long, society-changing, cultural-influencing twenty-year conflict, most signs of a battle-worn nation were all, bar few, gone. Luckily for me, enabling me to feed my Vietnamese-renamed-and-reclaimed American War interest, the remaining scar-bearing places had been transformed into tourist attractions with guides enthusiastically describing battles between American soldiers and the Viet Cong, pointing out ancient temples damaged by air attacks.

At the Củ Chi tunnels, where I collapsed, visitors can crawl through some of the elaborate underground tunnels built during the war to house the locals, escape attacks and ambush the unexpected enemy. Also, for a small fee, gung-ho tourists are given the opportunity to satisfy their own military combat desires by shooting firearms used during the war.

Unfortunately, I didn't quite get to properly experience the Củ Chi tunnels. My brain had other ideas.

Throughout the history of Vietnam, it had always been under threat of attack from other dominating nations. Their neighbour China fought to possess their fertile land for over a thousand years.

The French ruled for close to a hundred years, hence why the hospital I stayed in was named Franco Vasco with all the French doctors, Napoleon and the Revolution. And then there was the American War. Surprisingly, after all that repression, the Vietnamese people formed one of the happiest and friendliest cultures I had ever met throughout my travels.

We first touched down at Nội Bài International Airport in the country's north, about an hour from the city of Hanoi. It was nearing midnight on Saturday, March 28, 2009, nine days prior to D-day. Our itinerary was to spend about five days in the northern region, then head south-central along the east coast for some chill time, and then move on to Ho Chi Minh City (Saigon) for the remainder of our trip.

No matter how many times I visit Asia, the way people drive there never fails to bring out the 'nervous nanna on a caffeine rush' in me. It's the first thing everyone who visits will notice. No travel vaccine will protect you from the madness. It's practically a 'Welcome to the Far East' arrival greeting, injected with a shot of adrenaline. The irony is that Asia is a place renowned for its humble spiritual understanding, the world's karmic heartbeat, a tranquil haven of religious serenity.

But not on the roads! It's one for all, all for one; kill or be killed, live and let live.

We soon learnt the rules of the road: there are none!

After a one-hour death-defying, dashboard-bracing, jaw-clenching, leg-pinned-as-straight-as-an-arrow-and-imbedded-into-the-floor-slamming-an-imaginary passenger-brake drive from the airport to Hanoi, any sleep deprivation we might have felt was left behind at the baggage carousel.

'We're here, we've made it!' My travel weariness was instantly wiped away by the thrill of a city thumping like a subwoofer. 'There must be some kind of festival on.' Tourists looking for a good time jammed the streets like strawberry marmalade. Locals pulsed through the Saturday night antics while swarms of motorcycles dodged and darted in between the congestion. A human ant farm at peak hours working overtime.

Sparkling like a bottle of Dom Pérignon, the old French-influenced northern capital was alight with shop after shop, restaurants upon restaurants, and hotels and food stores open at all hours, covering all trades. Parked mopeds were scattered everywhere like a pile of wind-blown leaves—on pavements, sidewalks, corners, doorways, lanes, here, there, anywhere—leaving no room for a casual evening footpath stroll.

With all the windows down, intoxicating air tunnelled through. Our taxi smelt like an Asian street carnival mixed with carbon fumes and tropical heat. Bursts of endless tooting horns blared like a siren, warning street-bound pedestrians to move out of the way.

Adjacent a construction site, amongst the mayhem workmen casually shovelled sand into wheelbarrows on the edge of the street as traffic skilfully squeezed through their undesignated work area. Traffic went whizzing in between bodies sporting no safety boots, no hi-vis, no hard hats. No sanity.

With one hand on the steering wheel and the other riding the horn, our driver nudged through the hive of activity metre by metre, foot by foot, dividing the ocean of people like the parting of the Red Sea as we weaved our way through like royalty.

At last we made it to our hotel, bang in the middle of the madness, right in the heart of the old quarters. Three stars of luxury heaven!

Our first night in the eighties-inspired budget sanctuary hotel was a restless one. The mattresses had looked a lot more comfortable over the Internet, and the glossary had failed to mention the giant rat.

It was early Sunday morning when we first emerged from our hotel. Still running on Melbourne time, the four-hour difference meant our body clocks required resetting. The curbside awash with litter from the previous night's chaos, the zipping motorcycles and tooting horns had since dispersed. Like a ghost town, the cobblestoned streets were quiet and empty as eager travellers enjoyed hotel breakfasts, strolled pavements and perused the streets.

Along the curb's edge, a rickshaw pulled up. 'Hello, my name Diesel.'

'Hi, how much for ride around city?' I don't know what it is about us Westerners—as soon as we notice someone's English isn't the best, we automatically break into speech minus pronouns, grammar tossed like an unfinished salad.

'No worry, I do good price!' We performed the customary contractual arm wrestle, bartering for the best deal. The cost of a pie with sauce for us, the price of a week's groceries for them.

A second rickshaw appeared out of nowhere—poof, just like that—to help accommodate the five of us. 'This my brother-law.' There's always a family member lurking in the shadows, watching from a distance. They wait on standby, available, inconspicuously burning a hole in you with their eyes, waiting for a nod of the head from their mate, and in a flash they're there to get in on the money-making action, seal the deal.

We stepped into the rickshaw's rear canopied bench seats, ready for our first adventure—Molly with her mum in one, Charlotte and myself in the other, baby Maddie on my lap.

'My real name Vin.' The man stood on the pedals, pushing through with his feather-weight body, trying to gain some motion. Elbows locked, hands on handlebars, he turned his head, looking at us over his shoulder. 'My name like Hollywood movie star Vin Diesel.' A novel marketing tool for potential customers, providing a sense of security, an element of trust—*If Vin Diesel can't look after you on this Hanoi expedition, no one can!* And though they looked nothing alike—our Diesel was short, thin and Asian—he had plenty of strength in those tiny little legs of his to propel that rickshaw for several hours. We were guided through the endless meandering streets of Hanoi, accompanied with a verbal tour guide in broken English.

'Tonight, I eat like king!' A smile of pride stamped across Vin's face, hunger in his eyes. Locked elbows, head turned as he pushed through the pedals. Like a weathered hinge on an old side gate, our bartering skills were a little rusty.

As the traffic grew to the intensity we had witnessed upon our arrival—thumping subwoofer, marmalade streets—the rickshaw offered us an unspoilt wide-angled 4K view amidst the congested madness. Smells, tastes, sounds and sights made our eyes water, drowning our senses. *Beep, beep, beep, beep!* We were in the jam, swimming in marmalade, immersed in the thick of it.

Motorcycles, mopeds, cars, taxis, buses and trucks engulfed us, squeezing through impossible spaces just centimetres away, millimetres too close. Honking their horns into a crescendo of noise while complying to the *'no rules' traffic policy,* they dashed through intersections, effortlessly flowing into streams of traffic as the other vehicles simply moved over, letting them in. No road rage!

New arrival pedestrians, foreigners, stood on the edges, attempting to find a pattern in the unpredictable current of traffic. Calculating when to cross, doing the maths, learning the 'no rules' rule. Breath held, bravely facing the unforgiving insanity. *One, two, three, go!*

Our first stop was a war memorial museum, artefacts from the aforementioned war on display. On the grounds stood a three-storey watchtower where soldiers had once kept a lookout for the approaching enemy, the Viet Cong. We climbed the narrow chisel-stoned spiral staircase corkscrewing its way up and around the tower's internal circumference, leading us onto the balcony. Views from the top stretched far across the grey city, the Dom Pérignon sparkle blanketed by a fog of pollution, covered in a film of dust, the presence of poverty everywhere.

To escape life in fast-forward, we stepped outside the population problem. Locals and tourists found peace at a Buddhist temple humbly nestled in between the chaos. We calmly walked through the still, fresh garden, lost in the moment, our mobile phones off and new experiences on. Tranquil moving waters and burning oils pushed the symphony of horns into the fading distance. *Ohm.*

'Can we take photo, please?' A group of Japanese tourists fascinated by Charlotte's geisha-like appearance, circling around her, framed her through their Nikon viewfinders. They were pointing, aiming and happily snapping, capturing the moment to show folks back home. She bashfully became the centre's star attraction.

Disturbing the peace, Molly—unable to resist temptation—banged the temple's gong, then took refuge behind me as the annoyed monk chased her away.

Maddie napped in her pram, jet-lagged.

Back in the rapid stream, our cycle tour continued, rubbing shoulders with the hordes of traffic. Through the city parliament district and past the government buildings surrounded by a tall concrete wall, military guards stood motionless in their honour to defend their nation.

I don't recall seeing any monumental landmark buildings that you would find in most countries. The French didn't leave behind an Eiffel Tower replica; there was no Tiananmen Square left by the Chinese. However, the city did have a certain pulsating attraction that kept you wanting to know what was around the next endless corner, down the winding alleyway, up the rackety street, keeping the excitement *thumping like a subwoofer.*

*Today, I feel like king!*

With his back to us, our movie star chauffeur smoothly pushed through the tricycle's peddles, knee up, leg down, casually cruising along. 'This big market for buy food,' he said, pulling the rickshaw to the side.

Aromas of Asian spices wrapped in a ting of putrid sewer scent spilled out into the street. Heckles of traders and punters negotiating the price of fish echoed all around; the chatter permeated the air like thousands of chirping chickens condensed in a giant poultry shed. No need for Diesel to translate—this language, we all understood.

Next was the alluring visual spectacle of exotic, unfamiliar fruit that filled the market stalls, drawing us in, pulling us through—*mobile phones off and new experiences on*. Avocados the size of a hand; bananas as long as your forearm. Prickly, spiky, oddly shaped multi-coloured fruit. Prices as low as three hundred dong, a measly few cents for us. Traders and punters chirping, heckling, *a crescendo of noise*. We stood shoulder to shoulder, limb to limb, *squeezing through impossible spaces*.

Further along, shocking displays of freshly slaughtered animals were laid out on collapsible tables, erected in the dawn of the morning. Dead carcasses were piled on top of each other, unwrapped, unrefrigerated, exposed to the open air, *the putrid sewer scent,* on sale for the public to buy. Recently captured fish still splashed in their shallow baths, frantically flapping about in the blood-stained water as we watched, open-eyed, our jaws slack.

Our rickshaw convoy progressed into the city's outskirts, peddling along the banks of the Red River that flows from southwest China into Northern Vietnam. We made a quick stop for refreshments at Diesel's 'family member's' tea stall at the river's edge, where we sat crouched on miniature plastic kindergarten stools, peacefully sipping hot yellow tea poured from a flask into small ceramic cups—*prepared in the dawn of the morning.* Our girls joyfully played with the friendly tea ladies. There was no language barrier, no inhibitions, the interaction honest and pure. Something truly special.

Apart from the continuous horn honking and engine revving rumbling away in the distance, creating an urban ambient backdrop, we finally had a quiet moment to absorb the atmosphere and feel the surroundings, blissfully thrilled with what lay ahead. I felt humbled to be finally traveling through Vietnam after a lifelong desire, and especially proud to share the experience with my girls. Somewhere different, *offbeat and not so obvious*. A happy and eventful day that kick-started our adventure of a lifetime.

It seemed common for all drivers to attempt to get to their destination in record time. Maybe it's a secret unspoken competition to see who can shave seconds off a two-hour trip and years off their passenger's lives, or maybe there's a yearly award, like the Brownlow Medal, for drivers who travel the farthest distance in the least amount of time.

Whatever it is, it's gotta stop. Seriously. Before someone gets killed!

After a three-hour white-knuckle minibus ride from Hanoi, we arrived at Hạ Long Bay in the majestic Gulf of Tonkin. A must-see destination for all visitors, and an unforgettable natural treasure.

It's impossible to avoid jelly belly when visiting Asia; all the precautions in the world won't prevent you from picking up a stomach bug. Only drinking water from sealed bottles and eating at reputable restaurants is the safest option, and highly recommended. However, be prepared, at the very least, for a little discomfort.

The first of the family casualties was our baby girl Maddie, and her timing—as you will learn later—was priceless. She started vomiting all over her mum just as we reached the entrance to the port. A surefire way to get everyone off the bus in a hurry and out of your way.

After a quick wash down with our water bottles, attempting to remove any evidence of what had been in Maddie's belly off Silv's summer dress, our unimpressed tour leader located our boat. 'Follow me,' he said, gesturing with a curled backward wave of his hand.

Shouldering a path through clusters of queuing people standing on the sea-worn pier, colliding with bodies from different corners of the globe—*excusez-moi*—our personal space was inevitably entangled with others'. The busy marina resembled the hordes of Hanoi traffic, dozens and dozens of boats all hovering upon the shallow ocean's surface, tied to the pier. Bobbing to the gentle roll of the waves side by side, we heard a constant *booffffff,* the dull thud of the boats knocking together, stationarily drifting, water licking up the sides.

With a raised waving hand, flagging our attention, the tour leader stopped before our vessel, our bus group eagerly gathered behind. As pictured in the tourist brochure, it was an old timber boat, all spruced up with a glossy coat of lacquer and some spit and polish. Scattered deck chairs sat on the sun-kissed rooftop, the meals area below and the cabins at sea level, all measuring up to the size of a Miami luxury cruiser without the mod cons. These types of boats are known as junks—appropriately named, I might add—but it was perfect, poetic, picturesque.

We watched the Frisbee launch of our travel bags from the pier into the open arms of the waiting deckhands as we prepared to walk the short plank onto the junk. *Heel, toe, heel, toe, heel, toe,* I thought, our arms suspended like a crucifix. It was a metre's fall into the murky ocean, with no handrail.

The pier grew smaller and smaller, moving farther and farther away as the junk forged a path through the pancake-flat bay. I watched till it became a distant spot, a speck of hectic activity left behind for a slice of silence, a piece of peace. I turned my back and looked ahead.

I felt my French fry lips, salty and crispy, blanched by the sea air crashing into my face. My eyes watered incessantly. We were pushing forward, gliding and wake trailing, the big-ticket item getting closer and closer: Hạ Long bay's natural treasure, a must-see destination.

I could see them in the distance, fast approaching, slow arriving. Soon they were right there upon us, an arm's stretch away. Towering, living up to the hype, some as tall as a narrow city building and some as wide as a bus, one after the other. Rock islands, all jagged edges, pencilled up through the water like they'd been shot from a seabed canon. Hundreds and hundreds of them all littered across the bay, poised, disjointed, random and majestic.

The Gulf of Tonkin.

The junk sheepishly sailed in between, canoodling amongst the spires. We watched the canon-shot rock islands remain stoically still as we drifted past, dwarfed by their demeanour, our breath taken by their beauty—a *narrow city building, wide as a bus*.

We continued to cruise deeper into the belly of the bay. Waves from the boat's wake gently rolled out towards the surrounding cliffside mountains, the jagged rock islands' ancestors cradling us in their open arms.

The deck crew busily secured the junk to the pier. *Booffffff, booffffff*. Our first stop along this cruise: a manmade floating island. A fishing village built on hundreds of large plastic barrels normally used in a chemicals factory, all bound together by rustic sawn timber carved from the mountain shoreline trees, hand tied rope, bolts and wire. They were masterfully sectioned together to form a series of piers. A marina handcrafted from necessity, sweat and tears.

The island housed accommodations for the fishing families, one- or two-room shabby-looking shacks that appeared to have been slapped together by a couple of mates and a slab of beer over a long weekend. We were privileged a sneaky peek into one of their humble abodes, sticking our heads in through the front door. 'Wow, look at that—there's even a television!' Shonky wiring ran to a sea-stained power point; a single ceiling-mounted light globe helped to combat remote living in total darkness. The energy supply was delivered by an old noisy generator, stored outside and tucked behind the beer-slab-built shack. A quick glance around the small room found some fundamental cooking facilities, somewhere to sit and a couple of bunk beds in the tiny sleeping quarters, partially divided by a patchwork of draped potato sacks stitched together with fishing wire.

Islands like these were consciously positioned throughout the bay. For thousands of years, generations of families have happily lived here, completely detached from society, self-sufficient, sustainable and resourceful.

An off-the-grid community. Harsh element immunity.

Unperplexed by their challenging surroundings, young children played along the decks, entertaining themselves, having fun and running around with a pet dog in tow.

A century-old lady sat by her humble shack, teeth blackened from years of chewing tobacco, her bone structure clearly visible through old sunken skin. Her extensively life-lined hand was outstretched, sky facing, seeking loose coins, a trade for a few happy snaps—*capturing the moment to show folks back home.*

Once the fishermen returned from a day out at sea, a dark morning on the ocean reeling in their livelihood, they'd transfer their captured prey into large nets attached to the pier submerged just below the surface of the water, an eco-friendly fish farm. The assorted species were then nurtured and grown until they were of a profitable size to sell at city markets or large enough to feed the family.

To prevent the island village from floating away, they were securely tied to the shore, fastened to solid rock. The ropes danced across the water's surface, pulling so tight they looked ready to snap, like an overstretched elastic band.

The jagged rock islands we first saw were, without a doubt, breathtaking. *It can't get much better than this,* I thought, and though the fishing villages weren't exactly a visual delight, the lengths these people had gone to just to survive blew my mind like a champagne cork.

Dom Pérignon.

My calves burned from the steep climb. We followed the winding paths in churning steps, hugging the mountainside as we ascended to the entrance. The extra ten kilos of my little chunk of love, Maddie, enjoying the view upon my shoulders further tested my endurance.

The temperature immediately dropped upon entering the cave. Flickering sunlight danced in through the opening, illuminating surfaces with colours so varied, so vibrant. The walls were smooth as glass, appearing artificial, manmade, like a magic fairyland. The ceilings were thirty metres high, the spaces forty meters long. Paths had been strategically carved by thousands of feet over years and years of curious treading.

Through a passageway and into a second chamber, we spied the serene castle. The girls ran free, squealing, laughing and happy, their voices ricocheting off the glistening walls and bouncing from the sky-high ceilings. A cathedral's echo, echo, echo.

Reflections from the bay's water shone vivaciously across the cave's surfaces. Marble rock formations that resembled various animals seemingly came alive—a howling wolf, a wild boar. According to local legend, the cave was named Sung Sot, 'cave of awe,' from the awe-stricken reaction of the visitors.

The postcard view of the bay from the cave balcony, high above sea level, was spectacular. *It just keeps getting better.* We could see the rugged mountain face cascading into the gulf's liquid emerald surface, anchored junks *stationarily drifting*, the scattered gothic rock islands from seabed canons.

Magnificent!

Before we settled in for a relaxing evening, floating in the belly of the bay and cradled by the cliffside's open arms, awaiting a moonlit scenic dinner, our final stop along this splendid cruise was for a little leisurely late afternoon fun.

Like a four-year-old learning to ride a bike, wobbly and unsure, Charlotte and I stepped into the kayak, squeezing ourselves in. With the end of my oar, I pushed us away from the pier.

'Charlotte, keep in time with me, nice and easy.' Our rhythm was as sloppy as a drunken drummer at a New Year's Eve party. 'Just relax, hun, I'll do the rowing.'

'But Dad, I wanna do it, too.'

Disturbing the sleeping water, we traversed across the surface, eventually finding our rowing groove. Jagged-edged rock islands were soon an arm's length away, *poised, disjointed, random and majestic.* Narrow inlets axed into the mountain side, beckoning us to enter, inviting us in. Just Charlotte and I, alone, dwarfed. Canopies of counter-levered rock cliffs suspended over the water, metres above the surface. They seemed to call to us to explore, duck beneath and paddle through, shadowed from the sun. *Left, right, left, right.* 'Hun, look at all the fish!' The sea life was swooning below our kayak, crossing from one side to the other, a rainbow of colours.

The silence on the water was immensely calming, mediative. The sheer enormity of the mountain face made us feel like we were intruders in its vast ocean garden, hundreds of miles from our regular lives, in complete awe, *Sung Sot,* of our surroundings. This is the last memory I have of one-on-one time with my firstborn as an able-bodied father.

'Dad, I don't feel well ... my belly hurts.'

I began rowing faster.

'Dad, I think I'm going to—'

Charlotte, casualty number two.

After another land-speed-record ride back to the three-star luxury haven in Hanoi, years off our lives cleanly shaven, we were all ready to hurl—to drive the porcelain bus. Geronimo! Racing up the stairs to our room—three-star, so no lift—the girls protested, 'Quick, quick open the door!' while I scrambled to get the key in the lock—three-star, so no card swipe slot. Desperately holding it in, our lips were tightly shut, stomachs turning.

The door swung open. We all pounced on through but suddenly stopped, frozen. There he was, sitting there, waiting for us to get back, our furry little friend.

The giant rat.

TWELVE

# The Girl in the Picture

Central Vietnam, the nation's spiritual holy ground. Rolling hills that echoed the practices of Buddhism, Taoism, Confucianism and Christianity. A place where you can lose yourself in the silence and find yourself in its serenity.

Humble forgotten villages sprawled across luscious green meadows where farmers harvest rice and children run free among wild gardens. Unspoilt.

Included in the central region area are three UNESCO World Heritage sites (United Nations Educational, Science and Cultural Organisation): 1) the Imperial City of Hue, with its temples, tombs, palaces, pagodas, and whatever else is still standing after the you-know-what, 2) the ancient ruins of Mỹ Sơn that have since withered away, almost completely flattened by air attacks, and 3) the quaint, architecturally splendid little town of Hội An, where we stayed.

During the war, the US military established a demilitarized zone (DMZ) along Highway 9. Spanning east to west across central Vietnam, it sliced the nation in two: North and South Vietnam, the rival sides. The DMZ was a series of combat zones set up along all the main arteries heading from north to south in an attempt to cut the artillery supply route of the enemy. And though the combat zones became the most militarised areas in the world, the armoured wall of defence wasn't enough to distinguish the valuable home-ground advantage of the North Vietnamese.

Sheer determination of the underdog led them to carve elaborate trails through the jungle terrain. They hacked paths into the dense forest, cut through the combat zones and fought to raise the reins of repression. A justification for all the deaths.

Some of the most controversial and bloodiest battles through the entire war had taken place at the DMZ sites, resulting in thousands upon thousands of lives brutally lost. Horrific video footage was telecast across the globe and into people's homes, displaying burning villages, young children on fire and families scrambling for safety.

It was the world's awakening, a changing of minds. People stopped believing in the reason of the war, and more to the point, people stopped believing in the Western world's involvement.

Anti-war protests began. Demonstrations were held across the globe. Prominent social figures got involved such as John Lennon, Mohamed Ali. One hundred thousand people gathered at Washington's Lincoln Memorial, demanding that troops be removed from Vietnam, marching for peace—changing society. Flower power.

It was the war that shaped a generation.

Khe Sanh, a name made famous by legendary Aussie rockers Cold Chisel, was a small city south of the DMZ area, and the location of a US combat base. One of the bloodiest battles of the entire war, a seventy-seven-day siege, took place in this quiet country town. Sleepy hillsides were destroyed by endless bombing, caked with napalm and poisoned by Agent Orange, killing ten thousand North Vietnamese troops, five hundred Americans and countless innocent civilians in the process. A blood bath of young men, a field of disused souls, never to return loved ones.

And as we walked through the vibrant green grounds of Mỹ Sơn, perusing the ancient Hindi temples, some were ruined by B-52s carpet-bombing the region; others had been decaying over hundreds of years, decomposing, forgotten yet remembered. One of the few battle-worn places left to see had been transformed into a tourist attraction, with guides describing battles between American soldiers and the Viet Cong. They'd point out temples flattened by air raids, bomb craters in the earth and, to add some nostalgia, the army vehicles shuttling people from the visitor's car park to what once were battlegrounds.

'The plane come over hill and drop bomb everywhere,' the tour guide said, standing firm, proud. My eyes followed his pointing finger over the peaceful, luscious green mountainside. It was hard to imagine.

Whether his pride was genuine or if he was just following scripted orders, I couldn't tell. But the simple fact remains: The Viet Cong won a battle against the world's fiercest nations, whose armies used the deadliest war machinery available, and won using only guerrilla warfare, guts and perseverance.

And that's something to be proud of!

Potentially having your toes decapitated by a moped should be an official government travel warning when visiting Vietnam—*malaria, yellow fever and toe amputation.*

After the craziness of Hanoi, careless jaywalking was at the top of our 'Things to Do in Hội An' list. Closely followed by securing some rat-less respite at an impressive resort-style hotel where, gladly, our furry little Hanoi friend's long-distant cousin—*there's always a family member lurking*—wasn't getting a key to our room.

We had five days of lapping it up, allowing us to unwind like thread from a spool, a reprieve from the marmalade city. Every corner of this charming small riverside town was reachable on foot. China's influence noodled throughout the place like a stir fry. Colourful paper lanterns dangled from wire, strung high across the horse cart-width streets. They flowed from one building to the other on the opposite side of the road and lit up at night, glimmering upon a fusion of French and Japanese facades, an eclectic blend of sixteenth century architecture and wooden shop fronts, pretty as a picture. If you were blindfolded, then Google pin dropped right in the middle of Hội An, you would never guess you were in Vietnam.

Like children on a mystery tour, following whichever path looked most appealing was our prerogative. We ventured down laneways and along streets into openings, shops, craft stores and art galleries—no directions, no map, just wandering.

Across the town on foot in no time, our aimless wandering soon unfolded into a massive market tent. A lifeline of activity hugged the fringes of this heritage listed settlement. Canopies of tarpaulins stretched over eight-foot bamboo poles fastened in the flanks and tied to timber-wedged pegs. The breathless canvas tent contained the heat like a hot air balloon.

Sweaty palms, hands linked, keeping our girls tucked to our sides as we pushed through gatherings of village locals. Mums doing the groceries, stall owners shouting out specials for fruit, fish and meat. The town's supermarket; our adventure playground.

Scattered across the township like a tossed deck of cards, a saturated spread of confetti, were a multitude of clothing stores. *'Wait till you get to Hội An,'* we often heard. *'You can have clothes made to order for a quarter of the price!'*

Like a spruiker attempting to lure customers in, young attractive ladies stood at the open shopfronts, greeting passersby, *'Helloooo, come! come look inside!'* Flexible metre-long measuring tapes were draped around their necks; they were always ready to measure your waist, the length of your arm, the size of your chest. *'Very good quality!'* they'd say, trying to win your business over the abundance of competitors. Their winning smiles enticed you into their crammed-like-a-mosh-pit stores decorated with endless rolls of material racked in shelves, standing in boxes or lying on tables. Cashmere, silk, thousand thread count cotton—anything you could imagine, all there waiting to be selected. Cut to the pattern, stitched together and ready to wear in a short twenty-four hours.

*'I make special for you, mister, look very nice!'* All styles were welcomed: formal, casual, contemporary, business attire, whatever took your fancy. Stacked on the counter were telephone-book-thick catalogues jammed with photographs of handsome models, pretty

ladies, movie stars dressed for the red carpet, and rock-stars in funky jackets, cool shirts and distressed jeans. Customers flicked through the images, found what they liked, imagined themselves dressed in those clothes—*'I'll have this one in grey, please'*—and before you knew it, the shop assistant would be crouched before you, measuring the inside of your leg for a quarter of the price.

As loose as an old greasy chain on a worn cog, lax and lazy, our final morning in this delightful village was spent lounging by the vermin-free hotel's pool. Bags were packed and waiting in reception, my neatly folded 'made in twenty-four hours' cashmere suit—objective: the Melbourne Cup—resisted the zipper.

While I was decked in a banana chair, the girls splashed around in the pool. Maddie took a nanna nap in her pram while her mum squeezed in some last-minute retail therapy. I sat quietly reading, nursing that headache I mentioned way back in the ICU. You know the one—this should refresh your memory: *The only thing I thought could possibly relate to my stroke was a headache I'd had several days prior. But it just didn't equate; it couldn't be that simple. I wasn't stressed or anything—Christ! We were on holiday.*

My *Lonely Planet* Guidebook was opened to the Saigon section. *'Things to see and do in and around Ho Chi Minh City: Mekong River, Củ Chi tunnels ...'*. The last leg of our trip, and the one I was most looking forward to.

As I read, sitting quietly and gathering information, making a mental shortlist of must do's and must see's, I stumbled upon the passage of text which was to become *some sort of feeble explanation for what was happening to me*: breakbone fever.

A mere splash in a Hanoi bath, compared to a Hoi Chi Minh City ocean wave. Intersections were packed like sardines on motorcycles, marlin on mopeds, barramundi on bicycles. At least forty or fifty of them stood shoulder to shoulder, idle, waves of carbon emissions upwards drifting, hazing. Green light pending. Adhering to the nationwide road rules, some motorcycles carried a family of four. Dad, the pilot; mum, behind him; the firstborn at the back, and the youngest on the fuel tank. No helmets!

Junctions of streets, most without traffic lights, met like two rushing rivers merging into one. The traffic somehow streamed together with a seamless flow, smooth, crazy, yet coordinated. Jaywalking, unlike in Hoi An, was not recommended, unless you were rebelling against government travel warnings—*malaria, yellow fever, toe amputation*. The best way to cross the street was to first watch how others did it, then forget everything you've ever learnt about road crossing. *Look left, look right, look left again?* Not here. Burn that idea and follow these instructions—wait for the smallest break in traffic, a gap of a few metres. Then set your target to where you want to get to and just go for it. Step into the stream without hesitation, cross with conviction and pray to God, even if you're a nonbeliever, that the traffic will weave around you, swallow you into its rhythm and then spit you out the other side, unscathed.

Praise the Lord.

Our first day trip from Saigon was another highlight, almost topping the incredible cruise amongst the canon-shot rock islands of Hạ Long Bay, Sung Sot. We arrived at a small village along the Mekong River a few hours out of Ho Chi Minh City. Our collected group of twelve or so multinationals boarded a small boat.

*Pitter-patter, pitter-patter, pitter-patter. S*pitting and spluttering, choking and chattering, the two-stroke engine pushed the rattly old boat along the muddy waters, leaving behind a snail trail that rippled across the surface. My eyes followed the gentle waves to the riverbank and into back gardens of *beer-slab-built* shack homes lining the embankment. Open kitchens, metres from the Mekong, provided direct access to the abundant free water supply. Women washed clothes, mothers scrubbed dishes and children bathed. A private little insight into their personal lives, and a poignant little reminder of how fortunate ours were!

We laboured along into a narrow remote section of the river. The galloping pitter-patter slowed to a casual trot, *putt-putt-putt-*

*putt*, loud and abrasive, punching a hole into the silence, ricocheting across the Mekong, then dissolving into the empty distance.

Nearing a short shanty pier, the boat made a gentle rugby hip-and-shoulder tackle into its deeply buried pilings. Bouncing back and forth, up and down, back and forth, up and down, it rolled along with the soft waves till they eased. Rope noosed to the slip and with a helping hand by the tour leader, one by one we stepped up to the deck.

*Flip-flop, flip-flop, flip-flop.* Our thongs clattered like a one-handed clap as we shuffled through the sandy path in single file. Swish-swashing tall grass bordered the track, directing us to a small sheltered working community.

Soon we were safe from the sunburn-in-a-second sun and under the shade of a steaming hot tin roofed shelter. Parched and perspiring, our water bottles offered relief. Like little lost curious sheep, we followed the leader through the variety of workstations for jewellery making, basket weaving, timber carving. Sticky nosing our way around, we watched employees seated cross-legged on the hard, dusty ground, chipping away at their craft—smiling, happy!

'Come, everyone, this way.' With arms wide open, our shepherd ushered the curiosity-killed-the-sheep on to another section. 'Come, come try snake wine.'

'Snake wine? What's that?'

'Try, is good.'

For as long as I can remember, my old man's been making homemade moonshine out of all sorts of ingredients. Lemon rind, potato skins, orange peels, an old shoe—pretty much anything, along with some pretty damn good Melbourne suburban Italian community award-winning wine. He's a proud Italian man, and that's what Italians do. But, through all those experimental liquor-making quests my dad explored, never had I seen anything quite like snake wine.

Resting on the counter, it didn't exactly look like anyone had ever drunk any. Seemed like it was kind of just left there to fester, used for very successful shock value. There were small snakes, long ones, fat ones, cute ones, and so on all stacked, dead and lifeless, in large clear jars, all curled up into a snakelike foetal position and fermenting in a juice made of ... I don't know what.

'Try, is good!' Grinning like a crazy man, our guide handed me a shot glass full of a slightly discoloured spirit. 'Make hair on chest!' Yeah, like that sold it to me. *He must mean make hair on chest stand,* 'chin, chin.' *Dad would be in his element here.*

Back out into the sunburn-in-a-second sun, we walked along a sandy path and onto another shanty pier further along the embankment. It could have been the same pier as the first one. I wasn't sure; it all looked the same with the tall dry grass, the Mekong and us beneath a spotless sky.

The scene was set perfectly, with impeccable timing—better than Maddie's. Smiling Vietnamese ladies dressed in fancy traditional clothing appeared on the river, standing in Asian-style gondolas. Floating beside the pier, they were ready and waiting to whisk us off on another adventure through canals of wild grass and rice fields, a Vietnamese Venice. We nervously stepped off the pier and lowered ourselves into the gondola's seats. It was me up front, then Charlotte, Molly, Silv and Maddie in her lap, and our silent female captain standing at the end. Her long bamboo pole was embedded into the riverbed, steadily securing the gondola.

I wasn't even quite sure why I was so looking forward to cruising the infamous Mekong. I guess it was a combination of learning about Vietnam at school, the many war movies with scenes shot along the river's edge, the great music it had inspired and its influence on the world. Whichever it is, there we were, at the pinnacle of our trip—*hundreds of miles from our regular lives, in complete awe.*

As we coasted, everything was quiet, peaceful. Just the sound of water being disturbed, parted by the gondola. I found myself romanticizing history, visualising the battles had along this glorious stretch of water. Soldiers treading through the muddy swamp, chest deep, arms raised, rifles overhead. Echoes of gunshot in the near distance, helicopters flattening grass attempting to land. The Viet Cong closing in on the enemy, firing rounds from the riverbank, shielded by dense shrub. A frantic scramble by the soldiers as they board the helicopter, ducking, bullets flying. The cutting sound of the propeller blades fading as it clears out of danger, gunshots easing to a silence, soldiers lowering their arms. Something I could only imagine.

Lives forever changed.

Punctual and precise, the hotel's wake-up call rang till I picked up the receiver. *'Hello, Mr. Iannella, this is reception.'* Light splintered through the edges of the blinds like an old gap-filled timber fence, the room airless, muggy, drenched. I peeled back the thin bed cover, put my feet on the ground and stood to face my final morning as an abled man.

*Line in the sand drawn.*

I don't remember all the details from after I woke. To put this paragraph together I had to close my eyes, visualize snapshots of that morning, sieve through the fragments until I could piece it all together. I woke the girls and dragged them upstairs for a quick hotel breakfast, then we walked the short distance to meet the tour bus. It was our final trip to the much-anticipated Củ Chi tunnels, the day prior to our scheduled departure back home.

Chister—remember him?—was waiting by the bus, clipboard in hand, ticking off names on his sheet. *Here, here, here,* all accounted for.

In an orderly, obedient manner, the humbly excited group boarded the bus, filling the seats like falling dominos, one after the other. But there was some kind of mix-up—too many passengers, not enough seats, and due to the fact that we had kids, Chister requested us to double up with the girls seated on our laps.

No big deal. Well, maybe not, but let's not forget the explicit detail I have painstakingly gone to in order to describe the way people drive in Vietnam. Sitting in a hot, stinky bus with no air-con for two hours that was being driven by a bloke partaking in the *secret, unspoken competition to see who can shave seconds off a two-hour trip and years off their passenger's lives* meant we were going to be tossed about like dice on a monopoly board.

Apparently, I was quite annoyed with Chister. *'It's not hard, mate. Twenty-four seats equal twenty-four passengers! You don't have to be Einstein to work it out'*—I might've said something to that effect. I actually don't recall any of that; it was Silv who advised me, 'You're usually the one telling me, "Don't worry about it, it's no big deal"!' Biting the head off the bloke who helped my family and I through that frightening ordeal wasn't my finest moment, but it just goes to show the kind of person Chister was.

We lumbered through the city, doubled up, at tortoise speed, slowly chugging along. *Stop, start, stop, start.* Chister stood at the front up beside the driver, a microphone in one hand, other arm stretched across the bus, pointing to the various landmarks of Saigon.

'This parliament house the location where Viet Cong take leadership and celebrate victory.' Chister's English was fairly good, the best of all the guides we had met through our trip. 'Vietnam is communist country, and is very difficult for young people to be free, do things they want,' he passionately verbalised, going off script. 'They think I bad because I have tattoo and because I thirty years old and I not marry.' He paused, taking a moment to think to himself. 'I better be careful with what I say! No want trouble with government.'

On June 8, 1972, nine-year-old Phan Thị Kim Phúc ran naked for her life after a napalm air attack on her village of Trang Bang. The world-famous photograph that captured this incident encapsulated the nature of the war; it left a scar on the world's watching eyes. Kim suffered third-degree burns to her back and spent many months in hospital recovering. Some of her family members weren't so lucky. Her parents still reside in Trang Bang, and while the village has been restored and lives have been rebuilt, the memory still remains. A biography about Kim's story has been published, called *The Girl in the Picture*. Kim, ironically, lives in America.

We drove through this village, along the same road where this horrific incident occurred. Chister pointed to the exact location of where the photograph was taken.

The bus tires made a crunching sound as it pulled into the Củ Chi tunnels' gravelled car park. I waited for all the passengers to disembark; apart from the driver, I was the last to remain on board. The girls had made a quick exit to get to the bathroom, as after a two-hour bumpy ride, they were busting to go.

I shuffled through my bag, getting things ready, preparing our video camera for filming, excited about crawling through war tunnels. I stood, slung the bag over my shoulder, and felt a strange tingling sensation tickle my palms. I paused and looked at my palms, clenching a fist. I opened and closed my hands a few times, gave them a shake and then the feeling disappeared. *That was weird.*

Vibrating beneath my feet, I could feel the bus engine coarsely idling through the steel floor. The driver behind the wheel, foot on the brake, gear stick in neutral, was waiting for me to exit the bus. We were seated up front, so the steps were right at our feet. Just as I was about to step down, a sustained rumbling noise buzzed in my ears. Again, I paused, gently shook my head for a second and the sound subsided. *What the hell was that?*

I stepped down from the bus, the doors closed behind me and the bus pulled away, taking with it the life I once had.

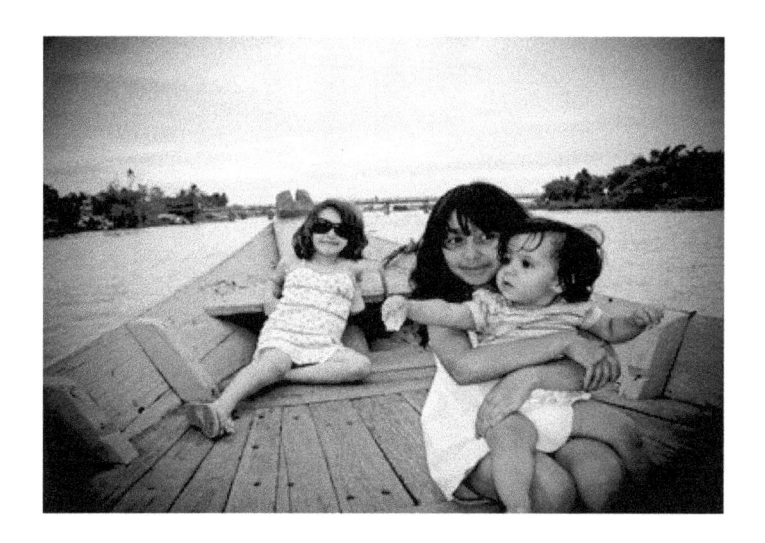

(Thu Bồn River cruise, Hoi An. Left to right:
Molly, Charlotte, Maddie.)

THIRTEEN

# The Severing

She stood in the doorway, defiant and determined, on a mission. Hand foghorned around her mouth, she was confident, loud, and clear, grabbing everyone's attention.

'Have you opened your bowels today, Mr. Iannella?'

TAFE, diploma of nursing, first year, semester two, the lecturer standing at the head of the class. 'Okay, students, listen carefully. It's very important your patient goes to the toilet every single day,' he announced. 'This must be monitored and recorded into their medical file.' Students were taking down notes—*monitored and recorded*—heads nodding. 'The best way to approach this matter is to ask them if they have opened their bowels today. Now, everyone repeat after me ... "Have you opened your bowels today?" ... Okay not bad, let's try it again. But this time louder! One, two, three— "HAVE YOU OPENED YOUR BOWELS TODAY?" Yeah, that's it, well done. Don't be shy, nice and clear.' Proud heads nodded. 'Also, class, you must shout this out from the other side of the ward, ensuring you use your patient's name so there's no mix-up. And don't forget to monitor it daily and ... what else? Yes, Fiona.'

'Record it into their medical file.'

For a second, I thought he was going to touch me. He was standing a lot closer than usual, his regular improvised jazz solo position requiring empathy, humanity. 'I'm afraid it isn't the best news.' Poker face, stern, serious. The Mechanic, the messenger of my angiogram results. 'You have had what we call an arteriovenous malformation.' Bonnet up, a not-so-greasy smile.

'A what?'

'Arteriovenous malformation. It's when the walls of tiny veins in your brain don't form correctly. The walls were weak and raptured, causing your haemorrhage.'

'Oh.' I paused. 'So, what do we do about it?'

'I'm not sure; that's up to the neurosurgeons to decide.' I hadn't thought of the Rowing Team in weeks. They were the ones overseeing this disaster, setting the stroke pace. 'The bleed has healed, so don't worry about it,' he added, wiping his hands with a dirty cloth.

*Easy for you to say!*

Like trying to siphon water out of a drought-stricken, dry-as-a-bone Queensland dam at the height of a record-breaking rainless summer, getting information out of the Mechanic, as you know, proved to be just as fruitful. My guess? Medical students were made to sign some kind of gag clause, not allowing them to elaborate about a patient's condition—*'It's for us to know and for them to find out!'*

The arteriovenous malformation (AVM) news washed over me without too much concern. Whatever an AVM was didn't really change anything. I had become so desperate to know why, thinking it would bring me some sort of relief. *So you're the culprit*. Like I could point the finger at it and blame something, someone other than myself. *It wasn't my fault—it was nothing I did!* Regardless of the reason, despite blame, simply put: I had a stroke, and I couldn't walk.

'Let's concentrate on your rehabilitation for now.' Probably the best advice the Mechanic ever gave me. 'You're very lucky, Mr Iannella!'

And there it was again—*lucky*. Said with all good intentions, optimism. Easily slotted into a sentence like a gold coin into a shopping trolley. Pushed in, chain released and you're free to go. It's yours until you're done, returned.

Though while I sat upright in my bed, cushioned by pillows keeping my severed string body erect, the counter-levered dining table wheeled conveniently in front of me and hovering above my lap, palming my tray of food as I attempted to rip open the bombproof-wrapped cutlery packaging with my teeth so I could get into my diced soft-serve meal—which smelt pretty decent—the word that sprang to mind to describe my eating experience was not 'lucky'.

It didn't wind me up; I could appreciate the sentiment. No harm done. But I kind of felt, without saying, that it was just said to fill the gap. A temporary filler to try and repair the crack, close the wound. To mend my shopping trolley's dodgy wheel that steered me in a direction I didn't want to go, left in a car park, abandoned, gold coin not returned. And besides, I was still in a headlock with everything I had lost, rather than counting the short straws of what I still had.

By that stage of my recovery, I had gone from being a stroke novice to Australia's very own stroke ambassador—self-appointed, of course. I milked Long Arm for info, siphoned the stroke dam until it was *as dry as a bone,* and she gladly pumped it out with a smile, pouring it through till my emptiness of not knowing was full, satisfied.

Now armoured with firsthand newfound knowledge, to pass the time during my 'stagnant marathon' recovery I'd attempt to impress the medical students that would appear, who were still drawn to me like a fridge magnet. I'd try showing off for a little entertainment, with my tenuous grasp of the brain's anatomy—*murdering the monologue.*

Then, I'd move on to fulfilling my self-appointed stroke ambassador duties, advising my visitors about what a stroke actually was. Fill in those blanks that most of us have or are too afraid to ask about because we're not sure, don't really know, don't want to know, or don't need to know because *'It'll never happen to me'.* It only ever happens to old people, a friend of a friend, someone you heard about at work, someone you know. Someone like me.

'But you're so young ... were you stressed?'

The often-asked question was my cue, my chance to let them know. To tackle my stroke awareness obligations, for their own sake: 'Stress alone doesn't cause a stroke!' By my recollection, my speech was in good form, becoming rehab's darling as I shared my firsthand knowledge. I had something to say, something important. 'A poor diet, high cholesterol and high blood pressure, accompanied with stress over a long period of time, can cause a stroke,' said, really, for my own sake.

Some visitors would tell me random stories of gold. 'My aunty Bob, her neighbour's boss's postman, Kevin, had a stroke'—*someone you heard about at work*—'and he's fine now, delivering mail again.' This would send me racing back to Long Arm for explanations, answers.

Those warm, fluffy-clouded stories about people regaining their normal lives were, at first, a little confusing. *Will that happen to me?* But I was also fast learning, at an accelerated pace, how the impact of a stroke is much similar to the property market ... it's all about location, location, location.

That pinkie finger-width brainstem where my stroke had decided to call home would, I dare say, be considered prime real estate. However, much renovation work was now required to make the house liveable again. And as I began to better understand the brain's complex floor plan, the reason as to why my house was so dilapidated became clearer, enabling me to acknowledge that Kevin the postman was, indeed, a *lucky* man.

To confuse us all even further, the therapists added BFG (Breakfast Group) to my acronym therapy roster. Our breakfast was to be had in the physio gym kitchen, most mornings with the other patients, to get some tucker into us before the real work began: fixing and mending broken bodies.

It was an opportunity to meet others wrestling with the monster, share war stories and compare notes, whilst simultaneously being an indirect therapy session as we relearned how to pour milk over a bowl of Nutri-Grain. Get your sugar rush hit for the day.

The initial thought of mixing it up with other people in a semi-social environment *rattled me like a maraca*. Trying to communicate, eat food, drink coffee, hear and talk amongst a group of complete strangers, something I had normally loved to do during my AS life, made me feel so unsure of myself. I was super self-conscious, faced by doubt, full of worry, concerns and questions. *What if I ... ? How will I ... ?*

These were all-new emotions no amount of therapy could prepare you for—fears a shrink cannot easily shrink. The damage done, eons beyond it being just physical, was delicately layered like a lasagne. Duke had my back, and Long Arm was my confidante, but these emotions arose so quickly, so sharply—*Gold Coast theme park ride*—out of nowhere, and often when my support team was busy supporting others.

'Hey, look at that! They're all like me, in wheelchairs.' That panic didn't even get off the ground; I never boarded that ride. It was all conceived in my head, in my knotted stomach. The breakfast group actually gave me a sense of kindredship, a connection to some kind of reality, though somewhat distorted and perhaps *eons* away from what's perceived as normality beyond the off-white hospital walls. But knowing I wasn't alone, that I wasn't the only one internally fighting this rechart demon and had people around me who understood, through *firsthand experience,* what stroke really felt like was an enormous help—*indirect therapy.*

One woman was the youngest one in there, not even thirty—twenty-nine, tops—with black hair and Snow White skin. Up on her feet and waddling around like a penguin, she was fixing her own breakfast. I watched her move about. It was awkward, rigid, like she was about to topple over. It was the first time I had really seen a stroke survivor, or more like taken notice of how a stroke survivor functioned, and I must admit, I was a little taken aback, *far out, will I move like that?* But at the same time, I was somewhat impressed, pleased she wasn't in a wheelchair. She could walk. *Hope I'll be able to walk too!*

Not brave enough to attempt to make toast in front of a room full of new people—the spreading of jam is definitely a two-handed job, and I imagined my toast frisbeeing across the room and landing, as it always does, buttered side down—instead, I opted for a simple cereal breakfast and a lousy coffee. Which I made myself, I should say, with Long Arm shadowing behind me, helicopter parenting. 'Straighten your spine, tighten those rib muscles!' I reckon the Goddess and Long Arm secretly met after work to rehearse— *Straighten your spine, tighten those rib muscles. And again. Straighten your spine, tighten those rib muscles. One more time. Straighten your spine, tighten those rib muscles.*

'I'll carry your cereal; you grab your coffee.' Long Arm placed my bowl on the table amongst the other patients, then manoeuvred my wheelchair into the empty spot right beside Snow White while I held onto my lousy coffee.

'Antonio, this is … '

Snow White's story goes a bit like this: She arrived home late one evening from work with a splitting headache, swallowed some paracetamol and went to bed. Early the next morning, the cry of her baby son woke her. When she attempted to get out of bed, her body wouldn't move. Her partner called an ambulance.

Rushed into hospital and straight onto an operating table, part of her skull was removed to relieve the swelling. Surgeons then performed life-saving brain surgery.

Seated in my wheelchair, I was tucked beneath the table, elbow to elbow with my peers. Close enough to get a distinguishable visual of the varied collection of people, and what resonated most about this fine bunch of folks whom had their lives gate-crashed, in a *boisterous Vince Vaughn fashion,* was a roulette wheel, a random selection of all walks of life. A colourful ensemble of race, an even spread of gender. And this final factor, completely decimating public perception that stroke only happens to the elderly ... age!

The clutch was pressed, engines revved. First-gear therapy slipped smoothly into second. A few weeks of the minutest-detailed PT and OT techniques, buttock shifting, and Hokey Pokey-ing and I had achieved sitting up independently, no pillows required. On my own, Pat Malone.

Suddenly, my tiny world got a *whole* lot bigger. Now that I could sit up, all I wanted to do was sit up. Therapy breaks—sit up. Meals—sit up. Visitors—sit up. Sit up, sit up, sit up—no more lying down on the job. I would sit by the spotless window eating my Michelin Star-less diced dinner, sit upright on the bed, or sit in a chair. Then I'd hit a brick wall with fatigue and have to lie down, lie down, lie down. Should have listened to the Goddess—'You better take a rest from sitting. You're gonna tire yourself out!'

My friends' and family's faces would light up with happiness when they walked into my room to find me sitting up. Their joy was infectious; I couldn't help but to smile, albeit wonkily. Left side curled up, right side drooping down.

I was given the thumbs-up to use the bathroom unassisted. I could sponge myself down in the shower, brush my teeth at the sink, and shave, alone, with a really sharp razor, like a grown-up, all conducted in a wheelchair and without close supervision by one of the Grooming Guardians.

Self-care duties, reassigned. One small step for man, one giant leap for man/woman/humankind!

A transition was beginning to take place, a shift towards hope, stability and self-belief. There wasn't one exact moment or one single word someone said, just small blocks slowly placed carefully upon each other, day after day, piece by piece. Building a solid foundation, walls of aspiration, something I could rely on.

In many ways it was the change of heart, the lighting of the flame. It was here when I felt like this—*'Okay, what do I have to do* to get back to normal?' I wondered, almost rubbing my hands together, thinking, 'Bring it on, I can do it.' It might take me a year or so, but then I'm done. Next challenge, please!

With all the close and caring attention I was receiving from everyone—family, friends, therapists, and nurses—that change of heart, that lighting of the flame, ignited a feeling of love that I had never, ever experienced before. It wasn't like falling in love, or the love you have for your children. It was more of a vast, open, unguarded love, and I'm not even gonna mention that word 'lucky,' because luck's got nothing to do with it. To me, luck suggests you did nothing to deserve it. This was a love that we had all earnt, collectively.

Long Arm notched my therapy up a speed, gave the throttle a little boot. All the butt shifting, torso swaying and slow dancing exercises eloquently performed by the Rock Goddess gave my core enough strength to support my affected arm, raised in the air, reaching for the sky in a frozen backstroke position while I lay on the physio bed. And even better, I was able to hold it there for a few seconds without it crashing to the bed. 'Well done. Let's move on to something new.'

Her directions were specific, repetitive. 'Long arm, long arm, reach, long arm, long arm.' I sat at the small desk, tools to retrain my brain scattered before me. 'Steady, slow, long arm, long arm, long arm, good ... long arm,' she said, instructions like a *Rubik's Cube*. 'Try to hold your hand steady and position your fingers into a *C*-shape, then place them around the cup and gently squeeze.'

Those first few attempts to form my fingers into a claw-like shape had a hit-and-miss rate of about twenty/eighty, in stroke's favour. My deformed hand was a foreigner, running on Vietnamese ICU time with no clue on what to do, how to create shape. It had a mind of its own, its fingers illiterate.

'I've got a question for you.' Long Arm looked at me inquisitively. 'When your baby is born and you're teaching them to reach for their sippy cup, are you gonna say, "Long arm, long arm, long arm"?' She laughed, ferociously, then told me this: 'Hey, you know there's been some reported cases of stroke survivors experiencing something they call "spontaneous recovery".'

'What do you mean?'

'It's when after six weeks, a patient's paralysis is spontaneously healed, returning them back to normal.'

'Really?'

*Six Weeks Later*

'Hey, what time is it coming?'

'What time is *what* coming?'

'Is it coming in the morning or afternoon? I need to know so I can pack.'

'What are you talking about?' She looked confused.

'My spontaneous recovery. What time is it coming?'

'Bud, when I heard the news about what happened to you, it made me cry,' said one of my work mates whilst visiting. 'We were in a meeting and one of the managers came in to tell us. Couldn't believe it.' Wow, hearing him openly tell me that almost made *me* cry. An honest, heart-wrenching confession—*this was a love that we had all earnt, collectively.*

'Work's so stressful, it just doesn't stop'—something I knew all too well about. 'We had to pull down all the brickwork and start again.' Must have been the same numbnuts of a brickie he was telling me about last time.

Clearly overwhelmed by it all, he continued to get everything off his chest, cementing me in place with home construction *shenanigans*, in great detail, for quite some time. Perhaps the hospital environment made it therapeutic for him, rehabilitating. But I soon noticed myself losing interest, not really wanting to hear about the stresses of work, how frantic it all was—a job I loved so much, a team I felt such a part of. Belonged to.

I'm not even quite sure what happened during that conversation. Up till that point, realising all that I had lost—being relegated to *a bystander*—was oh-so painful. But now, as he was going on and on about work, I suddenly felt relieved I no longer had to deal with it.

The Severing.

FOURTEEN

# Happy Feet

Down the lift to the ground, through corridor after corridor. A card swiping to open the doors. Along a glass-walled passage with a view to the hospital courtyard garden—*very nice*. Another card swipe, a short corridor, a locked door, a secret knock—*ta-ta-ta, ta, ta, ta-ta-ta*—a special password—*grey squirrel*—and we were in.

I had my board shorts on, ready to go. 'You wait here. I'm gonna put my bathers on,' said the Goddess without really thinking it through. *I'm in a wheelchair. I can't walk. I'm not going anywhere.*

It was as hot as an oven in there; you could have defrosted a steak in under an hour. The windows were steamed up and the water was toasty, and we were about to have our first hydrotherapy session in the hospital's close-to-boiling-point heated pool.

The Rock Goddess returned with her cossie on and an aura of determination. 'Okay, let's get started,' she announced, then wheeled me over to the hydraulic crane-like lifting chair that stood beside the pool.

Now, I was pretty excited about doing therapy in the hydro pool. 'It's very good for you,' the Grooming Guardians would say. 'It's like doing ten physio sessions in one.' But looking at the lifting chair that was going to transfer me from the firm, hard, reliable floor into the water didn't exactly inflate my dinghy. *Is this thing even safe?!* No armrests to support myself with, no harness, no handrail to hold on to—just a flat metre-wide bench to sit upright on and a backrest to lean against. The Goddess must have had more faith in me than I had in myself. 'It's okay, you can do this. It'll be fine!'

Earlier, all I had wanted to do was sit up, sit up, sit up. Therapy breaks, meals, visitors, sit, sit, sit. But now, as I watched her dismantle my wheelchair arms in preparation for the butt slide across to the lifting chair, I doubted whether I had the gonads. I just wanted to leg it, leg it, leg it, out of there ... if I had been able to.

She stepped in close, bent into me and braced her arms around my upper torso, slow dance position, with my chin on her shoulder as I waited for her familiar signal. 'Ready?' We had it down to a fine art. We'd practised the shuttle manoeuvre dozens of times, from wheelchair to bed, bed to wheelchair, wheelchair to table chair, table chair to wheelchair and so on, so on. 'Okay ... one, two, three!' All I had to do was keep still and play scarecrow.

I don't remember if we used the Bondi short board to shuttle me across onto the lifting chair. I couldn't think about much else other than to just hold on; there was a lot happening all at the same time, and my not-quite-right (NQR) brain couldn't process it fast enough.

Ceiling fans spun, attempting to circulate the concrete slab air, thick and heavy. Patients were in the pool with their physios while orders were barked—*raise your arm, lift your leg*—making the most out of the 'ten physio sessions in one' philosophy. The activity ricocheted against the perspiring walls into a sloppy mess of noise. Sensory overload.

I sat dead still on the chair, bracing myself against the backrest while holding on, for dear life, to the edge of the seat. I swear my grip was so tight, I reckon I left an imprint.

An assistant operated the control buttons to the chair—*left, right, up, down*—while the Goddess waited for me in the water, watching like a hawk, ready to pounce if I should have a Humpty Dumpty fall, put me back together again.

The hydraulics began to push the chair out and over the water, its crane arms extended like a sleepy morning stretch. It pivoted me above the surface, ready to be anchored into the pool. I was still holding on for the dearest of life, imprint getting deeper.

My dangling feet hit the water first. It was hot; you could have boiled pasta in it! I was submerged up to my shins, knees, then thighs, and soon I was all in with my head spinning as fast as the ceiling fans, thick and heavy.

Confused, disorientated, didn't know which way was up, I heard a voice. 'It's okay, I've got you. Just relax.' The Rock Goddess pounced, grabbing me and pulling me off the seat like a mother lifting her child out of a highchair, all the king's horses, all the king's men, putting me back together again.

The water was barely four feet deep, but it was deep enough for me to fear drowning. My unreliable limbs felt tied, bound, and I was unable to control my own body in the buoyancy of the water. 'Take your time. Don't panic, I've got you.' My tumble-dried brain was still spinning, fast and furious, time warped.

'Are you okay? How do you feel?' I nodded uncertainly. 'Take a few deep breaths. Don't worry, it's perfectly normal for stroke survivors to feel dizzy at first. It takes a little getting used to.'

Never in my entire life had I ever experienced dizziness quite like that. Even as she held me still, keeping me afloat, the aftereffect of the nerve-racking transition into the pool and the overwhelming intensity of the heated water sent me punch-drunk into a tumbling distant stupor. After a minute or two of deep breathing, the surroundings began to form into recognisable shapes—understandable reality—and as I arose from the rotating state of consciousness, like a reassuring voice waking you from a deep sleep, the Goddess's repeated words connected. 'Good, just breathe. Good, just breathe. Good, just breathe,' she repeated, the message getting through.

'I'm going to fit these floaties around your arms and ankles. I want you to relax, let go of your body and let it float free. Don't worry, I'll support you.' She stood behind me, hands clasped under my armpits as I let go and surrendered, drifting like a river-bound forest log. As promised, she held me steady—*as solid as a rock.*

'Can you spread your arms and legs into a starfish position?' Floating on my back, the water trickling at my ears made it very hard to hear. Muffled commands filtered through, gargled requests just clear enough for me to unravel into some sense—*understandable reality.* 'Now raise your right leg and rotate your foot.'

You could have thrown your laundry in along with a capful of OMO and gotten the week's load done. The simple task would send my body into a contortionist twist, causing a whirlpool of a current that catapulted my brain back through the tumble dryer for a quick run on high. Confused, disorientated, didn't know which way was up, until I heard the voice, 'It's okay, I've got you. Just relax.'

Somewhat acclimated, we continued to work through a variety of oh-so simple but oh-so challenging exercises. While still floating on my back, I raised my arms, lifted my legs, bent my knees, rotated my feet, gasped for air, swallowed water, did the laundry. My body collapsed, clamshelled, my brain bounced around in my head, I had mind-numbing dizziness, felt overwhelmed, panicked, rattled, exhausted, exhilarated—I think you get the idea.

Another nifty little dance routine the Goddess practiced on me in the pool had me completely baffled. And trust me, she had so many, it would have made the penguin from *Happy Feet* look like an amateur. This one wasn't a slow dance—no, sirree, it was fast, furious, almost violent. Standing positioned behind me, she wrapped her arms around my midsection in a bear hug. 'I want you to relax, allow your body to float free.' Her lips were perched beside my left ear, the command loud and clear. 'I'm gonna flip you over sideways, then back facing up. You just relax your body; let me do all the work.'

I don't know where the hell this woman learnt this stuff. It was bizarre—if you were watching from the sidelines, you'd think we were practising for some kind of peculiar aquatic wrestling competition, participants in the WAWC (World Aquatic Wrestling

Championship). But I never questioned her methods; I just let her do her thing, obediently following her directions. 'Okay, you ready?' Then, in a swift single motion, she flipped me like a pancake, golden brown, upwards and over, returning me to the floating free on my back position.

'Wow, that was scary.' She gave me a moment to nurse my flipped-pancake hangover.

'Okay, let's do it again, but this time I want you to lead the move.' Resigned, I nodded uncertainly.

We practiced the routine several times, and each time my participation increased. While she maintained the bear-hug position, I had to lead the manoeuvre beginning from left to right, projecting my left side up and over in a tumbling motion, trying to flip myself sideways and then resurfacing flat on my back.

Heavy-duty wash cycle!

FIFTEEN
## Six-String Heartache

Shining like a diamond, bright and loud, the quality of my speech rocketed ahead. But so did the volume I spoke at. 'Dude, I heard you! You don't need to shout,' said a mate.

I projected my speech like I was making a public announcement, without a microphone, to a room full of people. Like that moment when you're talking to someone with a raised voice over too much background noise, then suddenly the background noise stops, and you realise you're talking way too loud.

Well, I didn't realise.

There were days where kazoo sounds rattled around in my head, like my brain was grinding an axe, and then there were days my head sounded like it was trying to send a fax.

Gauging what volume to speak at was difficult. To me, normal felt too soft; soft felt unnatural. So, *LOUD* became my new normal.

Back at Royal Melbourne Hospital, the Rowing Team advised me that the relentless noise in my head was a condition called tinnitus—*common in people who have worked with noisy machinery*—and the Mechanic suggested I listen to ABBA, with headphones on, to distract myself from the permanent white noise slushing around like a 7-Eleven Slurpee in between my ears.

Tinnitus and my right ear deafness often turned hearing into a puzzle with missing pieces. Sometimes I'd get the wrong end of the stick. 'Antonio, have you opened your bowels today?' the question reverberated across the ward.

'Ha, have I milked the cows today?'

Bad habits develop quickly, so I discovered. With the double whammy hearing damage, in order to hear more clearly when someone spoke to me—and to avoid mistakenly asking about milking the cows—I'd turn my head to the right, aligning my left good ear in the direction of their lips, trying to get a direct audible dairy line feed straight from the teat.

'Your hearing will never improve if you keep turning your head like that.' The Goddess's fingers gripped my chin, pulling my head straight.

Some habits are hard to break.

My weekday roster was chock-a-block full with therapy appointments: three sessions of physio, two sessions of hydro, five sessions of occupational, five sessions of occupational assistant, one session of speech, one session of psych, woodwork, and breakfast group.

The diary pinned to my wall was written in secret code, a code even the great masterminds of the world would have had trouble unravelling. PT, OT, ST, OTA, WW, Psych, Hydro, BFG—it was confusing. Even the nurses looked at it and scratched their heads.

Thirty minutes each and every day was spent playing a mind-tripping guessing game with Houdini, Long Arm's assistant, as she pulled a variety of objects out of her little bag of tricks, brushed them across my skin, then asked what they were. 'Focus on how it feels ... does it feel rough or smooth, cool or warm?' she'd ask, drawing my attention to detail. 'Listen carefully. What does it sound like?'

I wasn't sure where to put my attention. *Do I listen, or feel?* That was the mind-tripping part. Normally when you're touched, you feel, but I didn't feel—I only heard.

'Keep your eyes closed.' With my palm open, *sky facing*, my senses searched for a clue, a hint, a miracle, while the constant *kkkssshhh* noise of my tinnitus kazoo buzzed in between my ears like an annoying bee, accompanied by the *ksh-ksh-ksh-ksh* sound of an object scrubbing back and forth across my hand, made recognition by listening a bit of a *kkkssshhhamble.*

'Sandpaper?'

'Yes.'

*I'm a genius!*

That was pretty much a guess; no sensations were really coming through. All details were dulled, diluted, like a tiny drop of cordial in a jug of water. Memory transfer lost in transit, undelivered.

Houdini continued to pull rabbits out of her hat, rubbing them across my skin. 'What does it feel like? What can you hear?' We did the Hokey Pokey and covered all seasons, summer, winter, autumn, spring. 'Is it warm or cool?' She stopped at various locations, crossing borders—WA, SA, arm, palm, fingers, wrist—as I took stabs in the dark, wild geographical guesses.

'A comb?'

'No.'

'A feather?'

'No.'

'A fork?'

'No.'

Scrap that genius thing.

Long Arm had me working like a dog when I should have been sleeping like a log eight days a week, saddling me with after-hours duties. 'In the evenings when you're resting, I want you to hold the TV remote'—she was wringing the recovery dam till it was *as dry as a drought-stricken Queensland summer*—'and play with the buttons. Run your fingertips over them and try to feel for the bumps,' milking it till the cows came home.

A bit of a softy at heart, but a task-monger at work. Occasionally, Long Arm would sit with me during mealtime and police my eating technique.

'What are you doing? Stop!'

'Yes, Sargent.'

'Hold the yoghurt in your left hand and peel the lid off with your right, not your teeth.'

'But Sarg—'

'No buts! Use it or lose it!'

Then there was the nut-and-bolt exercise—I can't forget to tell you about that. 'Only use your thumb and forefinger. Concentrate on gripping the nut and unscrewing it,' she said, demonstrating how to move my thumb, where to put my fingers. 'Keep it by your bed and do it whenever you can.'

*Screw, unscrew, screw, unscrew, then screw and unscrew some more. Got it!* It may sound mind-numbing ... well, it was. But Long Arm played the long game.

Eight-day weeks of working like a dog, no sleeping like a log, Ob-la-di, ob-la-da, Nullarboring, Hokey Pokey-ing, rabbit pulling, memory transferring, Swan Lake rehearsing, frozen backstroking, star reaching, *C*-shaping, finger bending, wrist flexing—I could go on and on.

*'Though this be madness, yet there is method in it.'* —Hamlet

My hit-and-miss rate averaged somewhere around twenty/eighty. But now, Long Arm's long game had bumped my stats up to a nifty thirty/seventy. Still not in my favour, but it certainly helped put another log on the possibility fire and a bigger smile on my rubber dial—*sunken at one end, but still a smile.*

'I'm going to hold up a card of a complete picture. I'll give you a few seconds to study it. Then I want you to rearrange the cards on the desk to create the picture.' After about thirty-odd minutes—*twenty-nine minutes too long*—of playing picture card mind games with the Duke, he wheeled me back to my room. Not versed with the airlift voyage, he called for a nurse. 'I'll see you next week.'

A few minutes later, my Grooming Guardian waltzed on in. 'Hi, Antonio, how are you today?' Back through the procedure we went—potato sack, wiggle wiggle, jumpsuit, ascend, dangling salami, descend, and onto the bed.

So then I was just chilling, having a little siesta before my next therapy session, just lying there and thinking, thinking, thinking. Weighing up everything that I was beginning to understand, putting the pieces together.

I had just completed Duke's lateral thinking tests without too much trouble. My speech was bulleting ahead, and my trembling irises had eased enough for me to capture enough sight to distinguish shapes, colour, ceiling fixtures and even read. All done, mind you, with one dominant left eye flying solo while my lazy right still waited in its corner for the bell to ring before it would come out fighting.

As for my hearing, well, it was still a bit of a *kkkssshhhamble*, but the Mechanic was right. 'Don't worry, you'll get used to it.' Massaging my audio perception with the likes of ABBA was beginning to hit the spot, 'Fernando.'

So, as I ran over all that detail against the knowledge of where my stroke had occurred—*location, location, location*—I concluded that my dilapidated house, bang in the middle of Brainstem Street, was the dividing point of my deficits.

Anything south of its undesired address—i.e., my body—was in much need of some extensive renovation work, especially southeast. But anything north just needed a good clean, new carpet and a lick of paint. Sort of.

Initially, when those *six tiny little letters that make up one HUGE word* moved into Brainstem Street, *gate-crashing my life*, I was, as you know, in a pretty bad way. But you may also remember that *despite my present physical state, my thinking process, once the cloudiness settled, fared best after my stroke. Strange.* These were some of many thoughts trapped inside my head as I lay in ICU.

And as I was still thinking, thinking, thinking, measuring all that up, considering other examples, possibilities ... I thought, *How about my roommate?* He was much older than me. He was able to walk, slowly, and used his hands normally, but he couldn't speak. And then there was Snow White, waddling about like a penguin, awkward and rigid, who needed a walking stick and had absolutely no use of her affected arm. However, she spoke fine, thought clearly and articulated words smoothly.

The complexity of the human brain!

All that information bounced around in my head like a pogo stick, coming together to form some kind of picture and filling the gaps that were often left wide open by the doctors—*maybe, perhaps, we can't be certain*—and what I was beginning to understand, or at least believe, was how the processing ability of my prime real estate area was pretty much A-OK.

The problem mainly occurred when my brain tried to send the information and commands onto my body, heading south through the dodgy narrow neighbourhood of my brainstem, and that information, those commands, had no choice other than to visit my dilapidated house for a quick drop-in to say hello. Then, upon leaving, somehow the information would become scrambled, missing crucial components to successfully deliver the complete message to my southern suburbs.

Communication breakdown!

Thinking siestas were something I took often. It helped me grasp all the loose pieces of information and compile them into some kind of sensible order, to build an understanding, *some much needed foundation I could rely on*. And though I wasn't entirely certain if I'd ever walk again, what I did know, for *certain,* was I would give it a fair old crack.

It was through the thinking siestas that the Severing deal was sealed. I began to let go of a previous life I had so desperately clung onto, watched it slip through my fingers—*painfully discovering how all those things I had held so dearly in my life had now been hijacked, dynamics forever changed .... a bystander!*

The cathartic conversations with the Duke escorted my transition towards a growing state of hope, a solid sense of possibility. We thrashed out all the heartbreaking details: the moment it happened, the frantic rush to hospital, the ICU, the rescue flight, how I felt and what I thought. I talked lots and cried heaps. He listened, nodded, commented, and wrote down notes—*the Purana Files.*

And though I had already, and painfully, told the story a thousand times to my friends and family that generally began with, '*We were about to enter underground war tunnels ...,*' this often left me to wonder: What would have happened if the *HUGE* word had decided to Vince Vaughn its way into my life whilst I was crawling around on my hands and knees through those elaborate tiny tunnels? What then?

Telling the Duke of Earl all the gory details was like letting the horses run free, releasing the pigeons. *He had my back!*

As the positivity transition was taking place, my focus began to shift from looking behind me to all that had been *hijacked* to looking ahead at what I could reconstruct, reassemble. Salvage the best of a life and leave behind what had now become, through the Severing process, not so important anymore.

The flat-out-like-a-lizard drinking lifestyle that was just 'the norm' for most of us didn't fit my new outlook; it lost its appeal. I began to imagine finding joy in simple things. I looked forward to being there to watch Maddie take her first steps. Envisaged myself leisurely walking Charlotte and Molly to school, spending more time with the people I cared about and pursuing my creative interests that had since taken a backseat, put on the backburner.

Simple things brought me the most happiness.

Flashes of inspiration flickered, random ideas, thoughts and feelings that I would scribble down in a notepad, kindly provided by Long Arm. Some positive, many not so much—words, sentences, lyrics, nonsense. In doing so, another realisation dawned on me. An epiphany—I was now going to have the most precious thing we all have so little of. *Time!*

Time to do the things I loved, time to do the things I wanted. One of the very first things I decided to do with my time, other than rebuild my health, was complete a music project I had been casually chipping away at for years, but I'd *never had enough time.* And perhaps I hadn't quite worked out how I would go about it, how I would get it done, given my present physical state. But the thrill of the idea overshadowed the hurdle of the *how,* and now with time on my hands—or hand—and a growing self-belief, such things were suddenly a real possibility. *It's possible!*

Fielding in their usual slips position—*human airbags, fall barriers*—the two physio students stood, tucked at my knees. I sat on the physio bed's edge, the Goddess crouched before me, front facing, eye to eye. My bare ribs were basketball gripped between her *master puppeteer* hands, the imaginary love song softly playing. She swayed me gently, side to side, like she was nursing a baby to sleep. I lost count of the amount of therapy sessions we had spent just weight shifting, spine balling, butt clenching. It was endless—two, three, four, five months, maybe a year ... okay, I'm exaggerating. It was definitely weeks.

'Today, we'll make a start working on standing.'

Finally! Just what I needed to hear—a chance to get up off my butt and stand. And logic told me once I was standing, the next step was to walk, surely. *Reward me with rapid results. Within days, just a few physio sessions, and then BANG—I'd be up and walking!*

But there were no shortcuts. At least none the Goddess was gonna take, anyway. Back at the beginning, at our very first assessment, when she said, *'It's gonna take time, slowly, day by day,'* she wasn't lying.

'Place your feet flat on the floor, about shoulder width apart.' Now she was heel-seated, on her knees, right at my bare feet. 'Spread your toes and apply pressure to each part of your feet.' Her master puppet hands gripped my left foot, rocking it back, rolling it forward, side to side, spreading my absent-minded toes. She fanned them wide, one toe at a time, applying pressure to every corner of my foot, rocking, rolling.

Twenty or so minutes had passed. With her shins compressed against the cold hard concrete floor she patiently sat, slow dancing with my feet, a moonlight sonata. Back and forward, side to side, heel rolling, toe fanning, one foot, then the other. Everything had to be just right, perfect. She even checked the velocity of the wind by licking her finger and pointing to the ceiling. 'It's gonna take time, slowly, day by day'— never had truer words been spoken.

'Are you ready?'

*I was ready twenty minutes ago.* 'Yes.'

'Okay, on the count of three we're going to stand. I want you to lean your weight forward and then push up with your legs.' Bit strange having that explained to you, but I listened like I had no clue. 'I'll guide you, keep you steady. We're only going to try a half stand, okay? Raise your butt six inches off the bed, hold and then down. Got it? One ... two ...'

'Wait, wait. Do we lift on three, or do we count to three, then lift?'

'Lift on three. Half lift, hold, then down again. One ... two ... three!'

I gave it all I had, grunting enough to send me to the moon, crashing through the ceiling in a spectacular half-stand position, an award-winning pose. Feet apart, knees slightly bent, butt six inches off the bed. It was gorgeous—you should have seen it. I wished someone had been there to capture the moment on film to use the footage for a documentary about my recovery. Photograph the occasion for the local *Star Weekly* paper, front-page worthy: 'Stroke Survivor Stands Strong'.

By now I'm sure you've come to realise I've got a habit of describing things from a perspective that pokes the fun at those difficult experiences, the awkward moments—the enema explosion, man-handling Jamaican, tofu theory, salami dangling, Motorola flip-phone dude. Such is the great Aussie way. Often when mates came to visit and I'd tell them about what went on in hospital, they'd always see the funny side and make crude jokes, take the mickey. 'The nurse sponged you down in the shower? You lucky #@$%!'

Laughing with my mates, at my own misfortune, helped a lot.

Okay, so now for how my half stand really went: bent like a banana, half-standing.

Long Arm threw everything at me bar the kitchen sink. We played with blocks, beads, buttons and balls to the siren of *'Long arm, long arm, long arm'* or the regular mantra of *'Tighten those rib muscles, straighten your spine'* as I slouched like a teenager.

My left hand's skill set had been wound back thirty-five years, to the tender age of three, as I engaged in the terribly difficult and immensely frustrating task of inserting multicoloured shapes into the allotted slots of a kid's toy.

Everything we did, bar the kitchen sink, were things we believed would be extremely beneficial to my recovery. *I could see the benefits. It made complete sense; combining the physical activity of playing a guitar and the love I have for music would surely result in a positive outcome.*

For over twenty years, guitar playing had my heart. It gave me air, light and love, provided company during loneliness and a voice through sorrow. Up until this point, I had never imagined life without it; I'd thought it would always be there. Over all those years with my trusted ally, we had some amazing adventures. We made lots of music, did heaps of gigs and met tons of wonderful people.

When stroke steamrolled not only my guitar playing skills, but also my hearing, I was nothing short of devastated, flat and black like freshly laid bitumen. And now, a month into this *timeless recovery*, as I sat with Long Arm in yet another of many therapy sessions, the reality knocked me down further. Sitting there, openhearted to her wishful advice, my guitar nestled on my lap. 'Try and feel the strings on your fingertips.' My left hand wrapped around the guitar neck, my *lumped limb* throttling the fretboard, crushing the strings. 'See if you can shape a chord.' It had once felt oh-so natural, like part of my body. Shaping my fingers into awkward positions to form a chord, bend a note, strum, fret, finger, escape had once been effortless. Instinctual.

'It's too hard ... I can't do it.' The curvature of my guitar's body forcefully rested on my lap, feeling foreign. Not belonging to me, no longer an ally. 'I can't feel the strings.' Long Arm was silent, her face mirroring how I felt—like freshly laid bitumen. I just wanted to cry, *curl up into a ball and vanish.*

Six-string heartache.

SIXTEEN

# Perfect Blue Buildings

'You've been in hospital for too long.' I sensed a hint of bemusement there. 'Nobody gets excited about hospital food!'

Maybe ... perhaps they were right. But let's take a moment to look at those wild accusations from a different perspective—three square meals a day, hand delivered, with no need for grocery shopping, no cooking required, and no dishes to wash.

Not a bad deal, hey?

Yeah, sure, there was a trade-off—hot and steamy for lukewarm and limp—but still!

It was a culinary celebration, a food and wineless festival all happening on my counter-levered table hovering above my lap, ready and waiting for me to dig in. 'Where would you like to have your dinner, Antonio?' my Grooming Guardians would ask. Some days I'd feast in my armchair by the window; others, in bed. Wild times.

I'd gone through the tedious baby steps from spoon-fed soup to mashed spaghetti, chopped chicken, diced lamb, and now, hooray, hooray, normal servings. 'Non-pureed' meant dinnertime was finally something worth getting excited about. And boy, did I take great delight ticking those little boxes on the menu list when ordering meals for the following day. 'Whattaya reckon, bud? Fish, veal or chicken?' Visitor's opinions welcome.

Large portion servings, which I always selected, were never quite enough, a sandwich short of a picnic. No need to loosen my pyjama pants string to fit it all in; by the time dinner came round, I was starving. *Oh, man, I could murder an unblended Big Mac right about now!*

The hospital must have commissioned the CSIRO to conduct clinical trials to determine portion sizes, measuring and weighing every ingredient down to the last gram. They experimented with placebo effect foods, continental cuisines, and good old Aussie tucker. To confirm their studies, they also conducted a pub quiz at the local RSL to reveal the most common answer.

The inadequate food portion idea was designed to leave patients longing for their next meal—truly devious. It was the only way they would eat hospital food!

Attempts to discourage my family from bringing me things to eat was just as lukewarm as the meals. 'Dad, you don't have to bring me food! The hospital food is plenty'—not entirely true, but I didn't want to further inconvenience him. His visits were enough.

It was like an Italian deli in my room. Dad had *salami dangling* from the curtain rail, roasting peppers by sunlight on the windowsill. My sisters brought in fresh muffins, cakes, soup. 'You need to keep your strength up,' they'd say.

Soon, my lukewarm resistance turned stone cold.

What can I say? It's the Italian way. If all else fails, you eat! Italians consider food a remedy for everything. As a kid, if I hurt myself, fell off my bike, was hit in the head with a cricket bat or simply wasn't feeling well, Mum would say, *'Non hai mangiato abbastanzo! Mangia qualcosa, ti senti meglo!'*—'It's because you haven't eaten enough! Eat something, you'll feel better!'

'This will be our last speech therapy session.' ST was confident my brightest shining star was now match ready. 'But I want you to continue with your exercises.' I never really knew if my 7:00 a.m. vocal gymnastics bothered my roomie. He never said, his speaking not yet returned.

I may not have won the syllable wrestling title just yet; muscly words still required lip staging before I could tackle those monsters. It reminded me of the first time, many years ago, when I heard my three-year-old niece try to say 'hospital'—*'Ho ... ho ... ho ... tospitipol'*—but it wasn't as cute when I did it.

As my chin-wagging skills went on a lap of honour, waving the victory flag, conditions still applied. I wasn't completely free from the remnants of having a stroke-affected face, after all. All those cryptic analogies I've used to describe how my face felt—*feasting bull ants, crown of thorns, cling film face, rubber-band lips*—had merged into one all mighty Jackhammer Army, a united force, and perhaps during my recovery I didn't have those exact analogies at hand when trying to express to others how I was feeling. *'My skin feels so tight, like it's strapped to my bones.'* It was kind of hard to describe, unimaginable for others to understand, unrelenting for me to withstand. I assumed how I physically felt was displayed in the way I looked, but everyone was telling me otherwise, 'You look well, bud.' I was increasingly hearing 'Colour has returned to your face.'

All my therapy sessions were pretty much conducted behind closed doors in the gym or in my room and during business hours, whilst most people were at work. No one really got to see the painstaking details of the therapy exercises. Nobody saw my deformed fingers attempting to shape a *C* to pick up a cup, or the endless butt clenches, slow dances and bent-like-a-banana half stands we did.

I was now smiling often and generally in good spirits—grateful to have support, hopeful about my progress. Therefore, for most people, it seemed I was all over this thing like jam on toast. From the outside looking in, all was beginning to appear relatively normal and progressing nicely, and though Long Arm had become my confidante and the Duke had my back, having new inmate friends like

Snow White to talk to provided me, and her, with an additional outlet to express how those jackhammers hurt like hell to someone who was going through the exact same thing.

Snow White had several months' experience of dealing with the dirty demon over me; she wielded inside information about the workings of its devious tactics. In between our busy therapy schedules, we'd kill time hanging out and share what we'd been through—*let the tears fall as they may*—hold a space and provide support.

We became stroke buddies.

'The doctors told my family I may not make it through the night.' Her tear-drenched description of having part of her skull removed made me shiver. 'They said if I survived, I might be a vegetable.' A box of tissues sat in her lap as she cried, and I was in tears listening to her. I could feel the anguish; I knew that pain. But I was also amazed, a little envious and somewhat inspired. She had gone from *that* to being up on her feet. That's pretty remarkable!

Our dilapidated houses were caused by *different* reasons and were in *different* neighbourhoods, therefore the damage was also *different*—location, location, location. It wasn't completely all lost for me. I still had some on-the-improve function to my arm and hand, a thirty-five/sixty-five success rate by that stage.

Everything bar the kitchen sink continued. OT slipped into a higher gear with a quick one-two combination of fine motor skill exercises and some basic—easy for most, complex for me—household tasks, like chopping veggies, stacking dishes, setting tables, all designed to achieve two outcomes. Firstly, to improve function, obviously, and secondly, to adapt to life with a disability.

And though the purpose of the latter, adaption, wasn't on my radar—*as far as I was aware, I'd be making a full recovery*—the obvious was beginning to become clear. I was learning skills for life. Long Arm's patience was flawless, ensuring I gripped the potato correctly to peel it—*new skills*. Demonstrating how to place a plate down from a standing position—*learning a new approach*. Showing me how to button a shirt, tie a shoelace—*life skills*.

Through those exercises, neurons began to rewire. Axons started to regroup, adopting functional adaptions on how I would cope with a life as a stroke survivor. I worked damn hard following Long Arm's advice—I screwed and unscrewed that bolt, played with the remote, and all the rest with vigour, anticipating that at some point, sooner or later, things would kind of snap back to normal. I would have peeled a gazillion potatoes and opened a chippery if it meant returned function to my batter-buttered hand.

The therapists displayed a lot of respect for the power of positive thinking. They were cautious, selective with their words; they never made comments that could potentially hinder progress. *'You're never going to get full use of that arm, so learn these skills in order to make your life easier'*—statements like that would most likely stifle a positive outcome.

Aim for the stars, land on the moon.

The skill of a hand is the most complex moving part of our bodies. The detailed precision it's capable of performing requires thousands upon thousands of neurons racing back and forth, communicating between brain and hand, coordinating skill, movement and making split-second decisions. Considering the damage along our communication pathways, it's understandable why a high percentage of stroke survivors are left with lifelong disabilities.

An additional challenge to the already difficult OT exercises was provided by my disobedient, flying solo right eyeball. Occupying the corner allotment of its eye socket, it continued to cause crazy double vision. I'd often completely misjudge an object's location and clutch thin air. I could be looking at someone sitting directly in front of me whilst also looking at someone else, partially obscured by an extreme close-up of the side of my nose, standing to my left. My brain was still rewiring, regrouping, trying to decide which of the two split screens to follow.

'The stroke damaged your optic nerve, causing your double vision,' advised the hospital's ophthalmologist. 'Best thing to do is wait. It just may correct itself,' he said ... I'm still waiting.

However, I had my one good eye on the grand prize: walking! We spent countless sessions slow dancing, butt clenching and weight shifting, followed by dozens and dozens of bent-like-a-banana half stands. *'It's gonna take time, slowly, day by day'*—never had truer words been spoken.

The physiology crash course was taking effect; the Goddess had me convinced on the importance of core strength, core strength, core strength. Pushing me way beyond my very narrow comfort zones, she was triggering my deep abdominal muscles through leaning, reaching and stretching left, right, up and down while standing a metre away, her palm open, hand moving into various positions at alternative distances. 'Use your legs to help with your balance.' She waited for my shaky high-five, an extended touch, as I sat on the bed's edge. Earth's gravity was like a magnet, pulling my stroke-riddled arm to the floor with its weight of a dozen bricks—*fall barriers, human airbags.*

Executing a stand now resulted in a bent-like-a-ripe-banana full stand. But it wasn't just a simple voluntary stand; it had to be measured, calculated and concise, of course, just like an Olympic weightlifter attempting the clean and jerk. Feet shoulder width apart, spine straight, shoulders aligned, weight forward and lift.

Now, if you're thinking, *'Fantastic! About bloody time—at last, he's finally going to walk! Well done, Antonio!'* just steady on there. Resist dancing for joy just yet. Achieving the ability to stand up didn't mean I could stand *still*. That was another ballgame entirely; a whole nine innings of excruciating balance exercises were required.

The thing was, when I stood, I began to fall like a pine tree lopped at its base, and that natural sense we all have that tells we're falling didn't kick in till it was too late. *Timber.*

'Hey, bud, brought you another Big Mac. It's gone cold. Maybe the nurse could zap it in the microwave for ya.' Mates were champions through those times, my pillars. 'Dude, you can borrow my daughter's iPod. Hope you like *The Wiggles*.'

I could only stand aside, silently watching the *bystander* process unfold and take hold. They attempted to keep me connected to the life I once had, anticipating one day I'd return and be myself again.

But as I slowly began to let go of that person, that version of myself, I set the drinking lizard free. The Severing process at times did a pendulum swing between what was and what could be.

My attempts to piece together ideas intended for a new life spiked like a porcupine; shedding thirty-eight years of oneself is no easy feat. I was weighing, waiting and weighing every ingredient again, *down to the last gram*. Sad to lose touch, glad to let go. Sorrowful to say goodbye, hopeful to say hello. The fear of missing out, the joy of missing out.

Late lonely evenings were when the desolate wolves came beating at my door, barging their way in. Everyone had gone home to their loved ones. Doctors had retired their stethoscopes, therapists had left their patients unresolved, nurses were on quiet night duty. Visiting hours were over.

At night the ward bestowed an echoing whisper of heartache, a silent rumble of desperation. Patients—some unable to walk, some unable to talk, many incapable of both—lay on their beds in their pastel colour-schemed rooms. Off-white walls, withering flowers, top-notch chocolate.

Those empty nights punched through my spirit like an earthquake, a 9.5 on the Richter scale. I'd quietly speak to my dearly departed mother, 'Hey, Mum, look at me,' tears muted, *falling, cascading*. If she were alive, I don't think I could have borne to see her pain, the heartbreak. She knew firsthand what it was like to be ill to that degree. She had fought challenging health issues for most of her life, till the battle suddenly ended.

The memory of losing her brought forward to right now, in that very moment, zapped the warmth out of my room. It happened around four p.m. on a Monday, February 2005. I received a phone call from my brother-in-law—'You better get to the hospital quick, it's your mum'—his tone grey, flat. In a mad rush, I jumped on my motorcycle. *I'll beat the traffic,* I thought.

Zipping in between cars, dodging around buses, slow-moving trucks, intersections, roundabouts. Twisting, turning, leaning, yearning.

I halted my bike beside the entrance, kicked the stand down, yanked my helmet off and raced into the hospital. A nurse hurriedly escorted me to her room. My family were there, standing around her, sobbing. They lifted their heads as I entered. It was too late—Mum had already left.

My last paining sight of her was at the funeral parlour, days before the mortician's pampering, days after life had drifted from her body. We were given a private moment to see her forever asleep, heartbeat silenced, warmth evaporated, lips blue. Gone.

For a week, our orange brick family home was filled with distant relatives. Cousins, friends—*amici, paisanos*—people you only see at weddings and funerals dressed in dark colours, there to pay respect, give condolences, bring a casserole, a lasagne.

And once all the handshakes, hugs, kisses and tears had been shared and shed, our family home grew a whole lot emptier. Dad went to bed alone.

The heartache once again very much alive, burning through me, silhouetted along the dimly lit corridors, bouncing off the ward walls and into my room. Eyes closed, I was flooded by the image of Mum lying there, lifeless, on a cold hard table, awaiting preparation for her final goodbye.

My plight was made heavier by her absence. I just wanted one more opportunity to hug her, another chance to say those things I never said. To tell her how much I loved her. The words we all long to hear but find it so hard to say.

My silhouetting emotions had impeccable timing, visiting me after a punishing session in the hydro pool with the Goddess repeatedly flipping me until I was *golden brown.*

Penetrating, a *9.5 on the Richter scale*, the worry for Silv and the girls pinned me to the bed. My body, my brain, my stroke had turned their worlds upside down—*like a tornado ripping through a country town.* In a flash of a moment, a blink of an eye, everything changed. The guilt for what I had put them through was always lurking, hiding in dark corners, patiently waiting till my spirit was low, seeking weakness, vulnerability, exhaustion. With precision it would pounce, sensing I was nursing a flipped pancake hangover, resting my bent-banana self, then slamming me like the Goddess did in the hydro pool.

*Heavy-duty wash cycle.*

Foolish thoughts, I know, but I wasn't thinking straight. I'd just been body-slammed by guilt whilst in an emotional arm wrestle with the vision of mum.

The lifesaving determination and heroic courage Silv had displayed to get me home from Vietnam out of steam, momentum lost. Supplies for the treacherous journey depleted.

Mornings, afternoons and evenings all spent attempting to tame a tornado-torn town, provide shelter for the girls, stability, normality, led to her ropes breaking free. Unable to single-handedly retain its weight, the heavy trailer dropped its load, scattering all over the place, bottlenecking traffic as it tried to squeeze through and continue on its journey.

I had front row seats, helplessly resigned, involuntary reclined beneath the security of hospital blankets, cotton wool walls, the call button—*the bystander.*

There were times she'd turn up for a visit completely defeated, dragging the trailer load. A hollowness in her eyes, an emptiness in her soul, teetering on the edge of eruption. Crying out for support, understanding, to be recognised as a victim. My heart was waterlogged, guilt soaked, emotionally divided as to how to understand what she was going through, trying to see it from her perspective whilst grappling with my disappointment, my confusion. *I'm the one who had the stroke ... can't walk ... nearly died.*

I needed her to stay strong, to be brave like she had been in Vietnam. To keep it together. If she couldn't do it for me, then do it for our girls. They needed their mother.

Cracks appeared like bolts of lightning and ran incredibly deep. The eruption took place during visiting hours, painfully before others. Silv's ropes broke free, her load too heavy. No longer could she hold on, storming out of the room and away from the hospital. I can't even recall what specifically upset her, why she angrily left. It tore me to shreds.

When a relationship is thrown to the wall, a safe landing is subject to the quality of its foundation, and with long-eroded footings, our dissolved marriage lacked adequate cement to protect us from this *tornado*. Our crumbling walls provided no comfort.

I'm sure it's a little confusing. We were on holiday, all together, in Vietnam, as a family, as separated parents—being amicable. For the kid's sake, for all our sakes.

Our terra un-firma relationship had a ripple effect. Silv and my family had not seen eye to eye for more years than I can count on my hands. Just like those puppet strings, their connection was severed.

Through my recovery, *most of the available life rafts were being used to keep me afloat.* No lifeline was tossed Silv's way—*she steered the sinking boat alone. Aimlessly drifting.*

For a brief moment, this whirlwind we were thrust into had Band-Aid repaired our wide-open hearts, blinding us from the deep matters of our emotions, the entanglement of our withered love. A faint light was lit, giving our fragile affection potential hope that maybe we could try again, make it work. But crash-landing on decaying ground soon reopened old wounds, tender lesions that we should have left well alone, left to heal.

Hard to read the label when you're stuck inside the jar.

It's not like we didn't love or care for each other, but rather a combination of other factors that had massively rattled our structure. Insecurities, outside influences, personal differences, on, off, on, off, tugging and pulling, twisting and turning. And, I here now declare, I could have been a better husband!

Sometimes love is just not enough.

However, I saw that faint light as an opportunity to start afresh. To wipe the slate clean, erase previous history. As I was transitioning away from the devastation of stroke, setting sail on the ship of hope, all I could do was watch Silv standing on the pier of despair as the love boat departed from the port. Even as I lay on my hospital bed holding her hand, declaring my love for her, I sensed her reply, *I love you,* was strained with uncertainty. My hands turned to butter; she was slipping through my fingers.

It was a hell of a lot to process, way too much to endure. I had to distract myself, find little things to do to keep negative thoughts at bay. Sometimes I'd find refuge binging on the chocolates that filled my bedside drawer or flick through the channels on my rented TV and watch mindless sitcoms.

The thing that seemed to work best was listening to music. My hearing had finally adjusted well enough to understand what it heard. My brother Rem, a big music lover, brought me CDs to listen to, a collection of classics and a few more obscure artists.

One of my all-time favourite albums seemed to really resonate during that time, *August and Everything After* by Counting Crows. It's a stunning album, a perfect blend of raw beauty, jangly guitars and melodies that make you melt. The lyrics are gorgeously poetic, and the singer sings every word with such conviction that it leaves you breathless.

The lyrics to 'Perfect Blue Buildings,' a track from the album that I had listened to approximately 3,783,317 times before, took on a whole new meaning to me during my recovery. They felt unspeakably profound, poignant, describing what I was feeling in that Vietnamese hospital as I lay there motionless, blank, alone, while my kids slept in hotel beds, unreachable, only a few hundred metres away. *Somewhere in the middle of Saigon.*

My first out of hospital excursion required three days of prior preparation. I had to practice with the Goddess the reorchestrated Harlem Shuffle from the wheelchair into my dad's car and then, but of course, from the back of my dad's car into the wheelchair. Lord almighty, that woman didn't miss a beat!

The Mechanic advised me to watch how much I drank, as one drink would now be equivalent to ten. Cheap date.

Like Cinderella, I had to be back before midnight when the nurses did their head count or I'd be considered discharged, and my bed may have been allocated to a waiting patient. The curfew didn't concern me, as I would have turned into a pumpkin if I were out any later.

Convincing the nursing staff to coordinate my shower in the early evening was a tiny mission in itself. It took two days to arrange and generated meetings, group discussions and paperwork to be signed. 'You can't do that. We can't shower you at night—it's against hospital policy!' *Their finely oiled machine that had been intuitively developed over years and years cannot be altered; it can't be changed.* Good chance breakfast was going to come with a nasty surprise!

My dad's known for being a bit of lead foot behind the wheel, so I had to keep my head down and look at my knees during the land speed record drive. He'd make a heavy contender for the Vietnamese Bus Drivers Brownlow. Years had definitely been shaven off my life.

Other than lying on a gurney in the back of the ambulance during that assuring trip from the airport tarmac to hospital emergency room, this was one of the first times I'd been in a vehicle since. Seated upright in the back seat of dad's station wagon with his foot firmly to the floor, shuttling along, wheelchair in the boot. The view out the window sent me on a massive head spin, as fierce as the first perilous dip into the hydro pool, *fast and furious*.

Traffic flashed by in a long-drawn seamless blur, headlights blinding—*sent me punch-drunk into a tumbling distant stupor.* Houses warped past, enveloping into one another, a myriad of roofs colliding, front fences sliding. Everything was moving too overwhelmingly fast, too mind-bendingly erratic, and my NQR brain was working far too slow to keep up. *Just look at your knees,* I told myself, *and breathe,* remembering the Goddess's sound advice.

We pulled into the car park, and Silv was there to greet us. Dad yanked the wheelchair out of the boot and attached one of its arms, leaving the second off to give me clearance for the Harlem Shuffle, solo mode. The car door was pinned wide open, wheelchair strategically positioned, brake engaged. I took a moment to nurse my flipped-pancake-like hangover, quietly running through the Goddess's instructions. *Shuffle, swing, brace, shift.*

'It's okay, I can do it on my own.' Dad and Silv were eager to help.

I swiftly manoeuvred myself into the seat like a seasoned pro—yeah, I know, I rock—then Dad attached the second arm, swung the car door shut and shot off to park his car.

It was just Silv and I, on our own, standing in the dark of night and taking it all in for a second … a very long second. Our first daunting new configuration: me in a wheelchair, her standing behind. A reality check.

She pushed me up the wheelchair ramp that hugged the side of the building and stopped at the closed function room doors. It was quiet. Just the sound of traffic buzzed by in the background. 'Are you ready?' I was nervous, anxious, excited, swamped with emotions.

The doors were pulled open and bright light blasted through, accompanied with a quiet ambience of energy. The buzzing background traffic faded into the distance as my concentration became fixated on what was inside. All I could see were a few rows of empty tables, some band equipment, and decorations. My heart began to race, faster.

Silv pushed me through the open doors into the large long hall. Just as we entered, right on cue, like a bolt of lightning, a sudden eruption of cheers and applause exploded.

There they all were, a unity of people all standing together, at least a hundred of them—my friends, my family, my work colleagues, all clapping and cheering as if I'd just won a Logie. It was brilliant.

I'd had no idea. There were no hints—I just thought a few of us work buddies were getting together for a simple dinner, a night out of the hospital. But as I was rolled into that room, into a wall of applause, and met by smiling faces and greeting hearts, a surge of joy lifted me above the gravity of this tragedy and into the warm arms of a community brought together by adversity—*it was a love we had all earnt, collectively.*

There were no imaginary love songs this night, *no sirree.* I was fast dancing in my wheelchair, swaying from side to side, buttock to buttock, lost in the normality, soaking up the tasty sounds of the band—the last band I'd played guitar in—as they bashed out a few classics from the likes of the Beatles, Supertramp, INXS, Daddy Cool, and Aussie Crawl led by one of my oldest and brother-like buddies, who you'll hear more about later.

'Going once, going twice, going three times, sold to the lady in white.' By far the highlight of the evening was the live and hilarious auction—*'Hope you love your Makita battery drill!'*—a fundraiser conducted by two of my closest colleagues as auctioneers as they stood on tables, urging bidders to purchase items they didn't really want for three times their value.

In preparation for the need to use the bathroom during the party, I purchased my very own six-dollar urinal bottle from the hospital's inventory department and kept it in a bag tucked beneath the wheelchair. The idea of having to ask someone to help me use it made for a perfect antidote to stay sober. 'Hey, bud, can you hold the bottle while I ...'

Following the Mechanic's 'one drink equals ten' advice whilst most others had their fill of Dutch courage meant some of my construction buddies—Blundstone boots and hi-vis vests—generally had their wall of affection defence down. 'Luv ya, man'—I heard that enough times that night that it provided me with a lifetime's worth of bromance.

It was nearing curfew, and I had to get back to the hospital. I wheeled my way around the party and said my heartfelt farewells, hearing a few additional 'Luv ya, man's that would roll over into my afterlife. Silv pushed me out to the car park. Dad was waiting in his car at the exit, revving his engine, ready to bullet me back, and Rem joined us for the trip to home base.

I just wanted to go home with my family, to go home with Silv, lie by her side and fall into her arms. She affectionately kissed me on the lips, the kind of tender kiss I hadn't felt in years, then closed the car door.

Dad had another crack at breaking the land speed record, shaving many more years off my brother and I's lives. The emergency room doors rolled open, Rem pushed me through waiting casualties and up to the front desk, and the clerk made a call for someone to come collect me.

A security guard arrived to whisk me back to rehab and I gave Rem a big hug. 'See ya, mate. Thank you so much.' The guard swiped his card and the locked doors automatically swung open. He wheeled me into the belly of the hospital across tiled floors, along darkened corridors, and reversed me through swinging doors. I was floating, reeling from the emotionally intoxicating party. High in a state of affection, drunk with love.

For a fleeting moment during that short midnight wheelchair cruise, through sleeping wards and long corridors, I had a feeling in my heart—a rush, a sense, a knowing—that everything was going to work out just fine. It wasn't falling apart; it was falling together.

It was one of the happiest moments of my life.

SEVENTEEN

# The Interview

It was several years later when I finally learnt about the struggle, heartache, and pain Silv endured trying to arrange my difficult return home from Vietnam. Courageously keeping the battle to herself, she opted to protect me from the worry and the stress, leaving me to focus on breathing, resting, sleeping—simply staying alive, *ICU normal*. Most of this chapter was pieced together by interviewing her to better understand her side of things. Silv filled in the blanks and covered some things I wasn't aware of, and considering we were on this 'family holiday' as separated but *amicable parents*, Silv went to incredible lengths to successfully get me back on Australian soil.

Something I'll forever be grateful for.

This interview was incredibly emotional for the both of us. We had to take many breaks to regain our composure, dry our watery eyes and swallow our swollen lumps. And so, here I have attempted to interpret what took place through her eyes.

'Back at the tunnels when you stepped outside to get some air, I came out to check on you a few minutes later. You felt weak. I assumed you were dehydrated and suggested you drink some water. "I'll go get you some orange juice"; your blood sugar levels were probably low!'

'I don't remember any of that.'

'Well, that's when Chister rushed over. You began to collapse on us, so he and I walked you to the first aid bay and sat you on a chair. We didn't know what was wrong with you, then, within minutes, you fell apart.'

'Where were the kids?'

'They were right with us, standing in front of you, watching their dad crumble. A few of the blokes dragged you to the bus, scraping you along the surface. They struggled to get you on board. Pushing and pulling, bashing your shins against the bus steps. You were just dead weight.'

'I kind of remember that.'

'Just as I climbed on board with the kids, Maddie soiled her nappy. It wasn't a regular poo—it was everywhere. Down the sides of her leg, up her back and across her belly—*and her timing—as you will learn later—was priceless*. I was panicking. I had to clean her up, make sure Charlotte and Molly were okay and keep an eye on you.'

'Nice one, Maddie.'

'During the drive, you were slumped in a seat with your face pressed into the backrest. You didn't move or flinch; you appeared to be completely disconnected, on another planet. That's when I thought you may have had a stroke or something. At the clinic, it was mayhem. Somehow you mentioned you had been bitten by something. The doctor checked your foot, looking for the bite mark. It was madness. I tried and tried to tell them it wasn't a bite, you had a stroke. But they wouldn't listen, couldn't understand—none of them spoke English.

'The nurses kept interrupting me, wanting my attention, grabbing, and pulling me away, demanding to see our passports, sign some forms, I don't know—it was so frustrating. I was waving my hands about, speaking in broken English, worrying about the kids—thought you were going to die. Jesus. Chister was there. He translated for me, and finally the doctor checked you over. There wasn't much they could do apart from rush us back to Ho Chi Minh in an ambulance.'

'I remember being in a room, and my clothes were off?'

'Yes, while waiting for the ambulance you were moved into another room.'

'And the kids?'

'They were in the room, too, sitting quietly on seats. Charlotte fed Maddie. The girls were incredibly brave, cooperative, and helpful.'

It breaks my heart still to this day when I think about what they all went through, how afraid they must have felt. *My brain, my stroke,* changed their lives forever. No child should ever have to witness anything like that. They are remarkable kids, and they really stepped up to the plate when needed. Courageous young ladies.

'And the drive to Saigon—what was it like?'

'Absolutely crazy. The driver overtook anyone and everyone at high speeds, screeching tires, braking suddenly, throwing us all over the ambulance. I was petrified. The kids were seated in front with no restraints, only the driver's arm braced across their bodies to prevent them from flying through the front windscreen. You know how I'm a terrible passenger. That ride scared the hell out of me.'

At the time, I wasn't aware that Chister had also been in the ambulance, in the back beside my stretcher. He provided enormous support during our extended stay in Vietnam, helping Silv wherever he could and checking in on them daily.

Silv continued. 'The first hospital we arrived at sent us on to the French hospital across town, which was better equipped for your condition. When we got there, the doctors didn't hesitate and rushed you through for an emergency MRI.'

'I don't recall the MRI,' I said, 'but I vaguely remember feeling flushed when in the elevator and hearing mumbling conversation between the orderlies who wheeled my bed through the hospital.'

I don't even remember hearing the word 'stroke' for the first time. My memory kicks in when the nurse began taping the heart monitor to my chest.

'Again, it was very difficult to communicate with the ICU doctors. They were all French,' said Silv. 'With my knowledge of the Italian language and basic French, and lots of hand gestures, we just managed to understand each other. They told me you had a haemorrhage type of stroke. When I asked them would you die, they just shrugged their shoulders. "The next few days are critical," they said. You were lucky to be alive.'

That word 'lucky,' as you know, never sat well with me. Through my recovery I heard it time and time again, mainly from medical professionals. I just couldn't associate the word 'lucky' with what I had been through. Finding twenty bucks in an old jacket would be lucky. Picking the trifecta at Mooney Valley? Now *that's* lucky—or better still, winning the lottery.

Maybe if it was said with a little humour—*I'm afraid it's not good, but hey, at least you're not dead, so you're lucky!*—I could probably digest it better.

'How did you work out how to get me home?'

'The doctors gave me information, including the phone number to the Australian Embassy in Vietnam. After your family, they were the first people I called. I spoke to a not very helpful guy. He advised me that there is a company who could fly you home escorted by a nurse and doctor, but ...' Here's the BOMBSHELL! Wait for it ... wait for it ...

'It was going to cost around $100,000, and our very own government would not assist with finances. They were only there to offer advice.' A deep breath. 'With some further investigation, I found several companies that provided the same service, but for far less. In order for them to coordinate your difficult return home, they required payment up front. It was Good Friday back in Australia, so everything was shut. I couldn't speak to any government officials or contact my bank to try and generate some funds. I had to wait until Tuesday, five days later, in order to get more information.'

I know what you're thinking: *How about your travel insurance?* Yes, travel insurance ... well, umm ... just one small problem with that ... we didn't have any.

Did I just hear you shout out, 'YOU DICKHEAD!'? I know, I know—trust me, we have kicked ourselves many, many times. We didn't feel the need or see the point. We'd never had travel insurance for any of our adventures. Asia, Europe, the Middle East ... no insurance, no problem. What could possibly go wrong!

'We had to find a hotel closer to the hospital. There was no point travelling across the city each day. The hospital was in the suburbs, so there wasn't a main road full of restaurants for tourists, no information centre and hardly anyone spoke English. We were the only white chicks around! The new hotel was walking distance to the hospital, through some suburban back streets, and we mainly ate at the hospital cafeteria. Rem and I would take turns seeing you. They only allowed one visitor at a time and for only a few minutes.'

'I know you were all at the hospital most of the time, but I only recall seeing glimpses of you.'

'The kids spent many hours sitting patiently in the waiting room. It was extremely difficult at the beginning, especially before Rem arrived. The hospital staff prevented the girls from entering your room. I didn't know what to do with them. I was so paranoid about their safety and kept thinking of all those scary stories you hear about kids going missing—I was afraid to leave them on their own. Look what happened to that British child, Madeleine McCann. She was abducted while on a family holiday in Portugal—they still haven't found her!

'I had to speak to doctors, make phone call after phone call to arrange your rescue flight home, fill out pages of medical forms, check on you and make sure the kids were safe. While keeping up a brave face, somehow trying to protect those little angels from what had happened. Jesus, what an experience ... it was a roller coaster. I wouldn't wish it on my worst enemy.'

Anguish strewn across her face, she paused and took a deep breath, tears pooling.

'I had to explain to the girls that they must wait quietly and not leave the waiting room. I put the fear of God into them, telling them that they could be taken by a strange person and sold in the markets. What else could I do? We were on our own!

'There was an incident, a little altercation with the nurses. Charlotte and Molly came racing out of the waiting room wanting to come see you. Two nurses intercepted, stopping them in their tracks, grabbing and holding them back. I heard the screaming and shouting as they tried to break free, so I quickly rushed over. The girls were so scared, they were petrified. I gave the nurses a mouthful, unleashed all my fears and frustration. I didn't hold back and let them have it. They couldn't really understand my words, but the message was loud and clear. We were having a hard time.'

Listening to Silv tell the tale through her eyes brought me to tears. I began writing this book a few years after that dreaded day when everything changed, and with all the physical and emotional struggles I have had to battle through, I thought I had arrived at a place of peace and acceptance. But as usual, the unpredictable emotions that come with stroke often catch me off guard, and I end up fighting to retain a poker face. Especially during the early days of my recovery—the vulnerable period—where I began to ask myself, *When does a recovery period end? Is it when you are fully recovered, or when you're satisfied at where you have reached, or when you just give up trying?* At this stage, I had no answer other than 'I'm *still* in recovery'—and besides, it was *still* early days.

Silv's next hurdle was to, somehow, find the finances to pay for it. During our interview, unbeknownst to me, she revealed just how difficult it all was.

'I called everyone, spent hours on the phone talking to government officials in Canberra, crying and pleading for help.' She still carried the hurt it all caused, all the stress. I could see it in her watery eyes. 'I spoke to employees at the Australian Embassy in Vietnam.'

*My brain, my stroke, turned their world upside down.*

'Airline companies and agencies contacted me at all hours, wanting more information, more details, this and that. It was so stressful, I barely slept. Friends, family, work mates were all trying to help, searching for ways to raise the money, but we weren't getting anywhere. No one could do anything.'

Then, by sheer chance while scrolling through her mobile phone contact list, looking for anyone who could assist, somebody to point her in the right direction, Silv stopped at a phone number she only recently added to her list.

She pressed the Call button.

After her short, distressing description about what had happened, filled with tears, emotions, and heavy breathing, her empathetic local bank manager took a chance to help us out. He arranged the funds we needed, trusting that Silv, once back in Melbourne, would drop into the bank, immediately meet with the manager and sign the relevant paperwork.

*The incredible strengths of human kindness.*

Now that the party was over, it was back to the hard work: standing still.

I'd never mapped out in my mind the steps of progress required to walk again. Each challenge I accomplished brought with it new challenges, and each task I achieved presented new harder tasks. I had naively imagined that once I could stand up, the next *logical* step would be to simply walk. But in between standing up and walking was one critical component, standing still.

Without the ability to stand still for more than a few seconds, walking would be a disaster, and by now you know as well as I do that the Goddess wasn't a shortcut advocate. She never blindly hoped for the best or took a stab in the dark, an uneducated guess.

She hadn't earned her nickname for wearing leather pants and fronting an all-girl rock group. She was thorough, skilled, precise, passionate—*as solid as a rock*. Everything I needed her to be.

Achieving the ability to at least stand up—not still, just up—meant I didn't need to be air-lifted in and out of bed anymore. Hallelujah! I had nailed the Harlem Shuffle solo mode crash course for the party—*shuffle, swing, brace, shift*—which provided me with some useful skills to confidently execute the shift from bed to wheelchair on my own, *Pat Malone*.

Pretty cool, hey? You're impressed, aren't you? Keep reading—it gets better.

'Let's stand you up between two of us and walk you across the room.' The time had come to get a gauge of my ability, see what they needed to work on. Determine whether my legs had any walking memory left in them.

Like an injured footballer being aided to the bench, they shuffled me across to the open space of the gym. 'We'll take it slow, nice and steady.' My arms were perched over their shoulders, the Goddess and one of the students scaffolding my body upright. 'Okay, try to keep your steps smooth, one foot after the other.' The floor felt a million miles away, distant, hollow. 'Ready, and step!' I pushed my leg forward, placed the sole of my foot down and guessed where the floor was, where the ground began, *holding on for dear life* to my scaffold team. 'That's it, nice and steady.' My legs must have had amnesia, flopping about like fish out of water. 'Just a few more steps.' We walked no more than three metres. I'm not sure if you could really call it walking, though; there was no rhythm, no rhyme, an uncoordinated mess.

'Well done. That was great!'

'Really? Were you watching the same thing as me?'

'Don't worry, it was your first attempt. We'll spend the next few weeks working on your balance and getting your legs to move smoothly.'

Now that they had me on my feet, they predicted I should be walking in a few weeks if all went well. And believe it or not, a rough date was set for my discharge: mid- to late June, about four weeks' time.

To help with my independence and to give the bed with the hoist to some other poor soul, I was moved to another room, my own private sanctuary. It had a single bed, an en suite, a kitchenette—better than some of the digs I'd lived in during my London stint, and when I was being wheeled back to my room after therapy sessions, I'd say, 'Driver, to the Hilton.'

EIGHTEEN

# Cotton Candy

On June 10, 2009, my thirty-ninth birthday, I received the best present I'd ever been given. A gift that needed no wrapping, a gesture that required no words.

I took my first unaided steps.

I don't know if the Goddess planned it or if it was just by chance. As I stood between the gymnasium's ballet rails, holding on for dear life, something came over me to just ... let go and walk. I took ten beautiful steps, one foot after the other, slow, smooth and brilliant. The best ten steps I had ever walked, the greatest distance in the shortest space.

I stopped, grabbed hold of the rail, turned and looked at the Goddess. She was grinning widely like a smiley face emoji, the one with the cute rosy cheeks.

Two months—eight weeks, sixty-two days, fourteen hundred and forty hours—had all came down to this landmark pivotal moment. *I did it—I bloody did it!* I had come back from the brink of death to being able to walk again.

Sure, they were only baby steps, and you can bet your bottom dollar that the Goddess was now going to hammer me with new experimental exercises she had learnt at a week-long seminar in the mountains of Nepal. But I was ready for it. *Bring it on—nothing's gonna stop me now!*

With just a few weeks to go until discharge, therapy was narrowed down to OT with Long Arm and Houdini and hydro and PT with the Goddess.

Just when I thought we had covered each and every new approach to life's daily activities, Long Arm had more, saving the best for last. I was making beds, fitting sheets, inserting pillows into pillowcases, sweeping up purposely spilt rice bubbles, and folding and hanging clothes, all done from a challenging standing position. I even practiced the task of showering while Long Arm instructed me on how to stand safely. I know, it sounds weird, and trust me, it felt just as weird as it sounds. If I bent too far forward, she'd holler, 'Oi! Straighten up.' If I raised an arm to wash beneath it, I'd hear, 'Steady. Careful, watch your balance.' It was like having my very own showering coach.

Dazzling me daily, consistent and persistent, was Houdini, pulling all sorts of goodies out of her bag of tricks and brushing them across my skin until one day, out of the blue, SHAZAM!

It caught me by complete surprise. I was like, 'Hang on, hang on ... do that again. I think I felt something,' and sure enough, there it was: the first sensation I'd felt on my left hand in almost two months.

Fan-friggin'-tastic. Hello, hand, welcome back!

Suddenly, the whole spectrum changed, attention to detail intensified. Long Arm's simple exercises that I'd been painfully baby-stepping my way through on the way back to home base were turbo boosted.

'Keep reminding yourself to grip the cup.' It felt like I was trying to perform microsurgery with gardening gloves on, the information faint, fractured, fragile. 'Nice and easy, steady, slow. Now take a sip.' The added spillage factor to the dynamics of raising a cup of water to my lips and taking a sip required monomaniacal focus, conscious thought, an internal dialogue.

There was a lot to think about, lots to remember and consider. *Grab, lift, sip.* My face still tingled with the United Jackhammer

Army feasting on my flesh, cling filmed. The cup resting on my lips felt as foreign as I had lying in that Vietnamese hospital. My brain was unable to marry the simple tasks together: hold the cup and take a sip. The two behaved like arch enemies, not willing to compromise, not prepared to cooperate. My rubber-band lips struggled with the complexity of form in order to receive water.

It drove my brain into a state of sudoku, a mind maze. Add the fact that I'm a bloke, and you know how the saying goes—most blokes can't do two things at the same time. Allegedly.

Now, as we are on the subject about blokes not being able to do two things at the same time, I would like to take this opportunity to express how I believe this myth was conceived.

### *Palaeolithic Era*

Cavewoman: 'Hey, Cave Husband, while you're preparing those brontosaurus burgers, can you get the kids ready for a wash by the stream ... oh, never mind, I'll do it. You won't be able to do two things at the same time!'

Caveman: 'Yeah, you're right, Cave Wife, can't do 'em both. I'll be by the fire, lounging on the rock couch and drinking wine I made from those berries you collected.'

Caveman's Mate: 'Dude, you can totally do those two things at the same time.'

Caveman: 'Shhh!'

Rehab covered everything: washing, stacking and drying dishes, wiping surfaces and even ironing.

'Is it normal for the assistants to bring in their ironing from home?'

'No, why?' Long Arm's face was puzzled.

'Cause Houdini told me I had to iron all the clothes in the basket,' I replied, trying to keep a straight face. 'It looked like her family's clothes.'

'Really?'

'Yeah, I had to put my foot down when it came to doing her undies.'

The balance and walking techniques that the Goddess honed in on made me look like I was playing solitaire twister. While standing on one leg and leaning against a wall, I had to bend at the waist to my side and shape the YMCA with my arms. Then I'd go down on all fours with an outstretched arm and an outstretched opposite leg pointing in opposite directions—the week-long therapy seminar in the mountains of Nepal was getting a good run for its money.

She'd spend a portion of each session heel-seated at my feet, rolling my affected left foot through the motion of a step, trying to get it to remember what its purpose was through repetition, repetition, repetition. All while I stood there holding on to the rail, watching and admiring her passion.

I spent much time on the treadmill walking at crawling pace. I pressed ten kilo weights on the workout machines till my muscles were about to burst and took regular wonky walks around the hospital as the Goddess measured my time and distance to compare to the statistical standards of a regular person.

It was during a therapy walk that I noticed the sign above the entrance to the ward: *Acute Rehabilitation Ward*. The huge sign I had been unable to see when I first arrived.

I sat with Long Arm and ran through the checklist of what I wanted to achieve by the end of my rehabilitation program, the list we'd made at the beginning of this journey. A lot of those lists and tests were designed to help accumulate statistics, which in turn may help tailor better rehab programs and be used by doctors to refer to when asked annoying questions by annoying patients like me.

Although I didn't quite achieve all the items on my list, I was told it was *still* only early days and I was *still* quite young, so making a full recovery was *still* a possibility.

My age, an ally in this arduous battle for better health, a benefit. *Good to know*. 'You're still young' was often said, and what generally came attached to the advantage of my age revelation was that fleeting word that I was *still* trying to learn to digest. Lucky—slotted in like a gold coin into a shopping trolley.

Hearing that there was *still* room to move, improve, was as reassuring as a hug from your grandmother. But with the *lucky* bit, I'd just wonkily smile and nod my head in agreeance.

Statistically—oh, how they love statistics—recovery could take up to two years. It may have been the Mechanic who mentioned that during a grease and oil change. Once discharged, my rehabilitation would continue outpatient, administered from the Community-Based Rehabilitation ward (CBR) attached to the hospital near the hydro pool.

Long Arm continued to surprise me, covering absolutely every single aspect of life that one would not ever think needs readdressing. Nutting out alternative approaches to all daily functions, *all of them,* as she'd done this *'a thousand times before'*. We already had the 'showering traineeship' activity ticked off the list, so now she wanted to mentor me through the private task conducted *in the smallest room of the house.*

There we were, her and I standing face to face, governed by two claustrophobic walls, a door and a porcelain bowl. We were positioned like a pair of bashful teenagers slow dancing at a high school formal, a safe and respectful distance apart, separated by her six-month pregnant belly.

She confidently took hold of my track pants' elastic belt band, then guided me through the lowering process from a standing position and onto the toilet. 'Careful, you're pregnant—don't want you to hurt yourself!' I reckon I said that at least a dozen times while I was in rehab, which always met the response, 'I'll be right, I've done this ...'—you know how the rest goes.

Then I practised the lowering slow dance in a fashion that the Mechanic would favour: solo, on my own, no physical contact as Long Arm stood in the doorway, hand on her belly, feeling for a baby kick while *life skilling* me through the process. Allowing me to keep my pants on, and what was left of my dignity.

Through those two months—eight weeks, sixty-two-days—I'd lie on my bed alone, unaccompanied, night after night—*everyone had gone home to their loved ones.* I'd look back over the last few months in complete bewilderment, astonishment, remembering some of those adventures we had in Vietnam and recalling the joy.

Projected onto the green screen of my mind's eye, I could see the clearness of that spotless Vietnamese sky, the warmth from the fierce yellow sun, happy and friendly faces, canon-shot islands, the Mekong. I watched in wonder, awed, floored, my *4K* memory vivid and wild.

*I captured all those beautiful memories on film.* With a cold chill, I suddenly remembered. My able-bodied life was documented weeks, days, hours before it all changed, moments prior to the trajectory that sent me *hurtling into space.*

For a second, I considered it a good idea to watch that footage, to see me being me again, agile, healthy, mobile. *It may be a good inspiration for my recovery,* I thought. From the pier, Silv filmed Charlotte and me kayaking across the emerald sea of Hạ Long Bay—*in complete awe of our surroundings, Sung Sot.* I pictured that glorious boat cruise along the Mekong, the tall grass, the rice fields. I saw myself walking, talking, reporting, capturing my voice on film, and my last steps, as we entered through the gates at the Củ Chi tunnels, moments before I collapsed.

My heart contracted.

I lay there, uneasy, among there off-white walls, pastel furnishings. A concoction of emotions rumbling within—doubts, hopes, fears, happiness, sadness. A path forward was still not clear. I wasn't sure of what was to come, what the future had in store, what was I going to do with myself. *Will I ever work again?* I was still holding on to my previous life, the Severing process not yet complete. Work colleagues frequently visited, attempting to lure me back, reunite our team. *Mateship, morning tea bake-offs, long lunch meetings, construction shenanigans.*

I was now walking again, just barely, which made me feel unstoppable. But simultaneously it forced me to entertain the uncertainty, the unknowns. *Will I ever be able to be the father I once was?* I took great pride in being there for my girls, always making it a priority to give my children more than my own childhood gave me.

For as far back as I could remember, my mum and dad did like other new Australians and worked—lots. That is, until Mum fell ill with heart complications, which led to valve replacement surgery and a fake ticker keeping time beneath her chest plate. I was only quite little and have a very vague memory of sleepovers at my auntie's place while Mum lay sedated on an operating table, unconscious, her chest pried open.

That's when it all changed for our family. Dad became not only the sole breadwinner but, much to his credit, a carer for his sick wife, our mother, which also meant he wasn't always there to be the type of father a growing boy needs. And though I only have fond memories of an upbringing filled with large Italian gatherings and get-togethers, once I became an adult, I painfully discovered the thing I craved most through my childhood was parents who were present, involved, connected.

In hindsight, that kind of childhood—not that it was bad, it just was—was the catalyst for the type of parent I set myself to be. Available.

I could now enter the hydro pool like a normal person, via the steps rather than the hydraulic lifting chair. Yay me! One foot after the other, watching my feet as I held on to the rail upon my descent, I was cautious yet liberated, buzzing with achievement. No floaties or assistance by the Goddess required; she stood on dry land, instructing from the banks like a swimming coach. 'Hold on to the rail and do some squatting.' Invigorating!

By that stage, I loved being in the water. Not having to be hoisted into the pool and have my brain run through the dryer, a *distant stumbling stupor,* was a clear sign of how far I had come. I felt a wee bit humanised, confident, capable. The buoyancy of the densely chlorinated water reduced the weight of my affected arm, releasing the dozen bricks dragging me down—*drifting like a river-bound forest log.*

My heart desired to swim, ached for it, but my *fear of drowning in four feet of water* rang in my head like an alarm bell. Having uneven function of my body made my left side feel like an anchor, lopsided like my smile. But I was so proud of myself, so elated, that the simplicity of treading through waist-height water, unsupervised, weatherproofed me from that heavy-duty wash cycle.

Now that I was at the pointy end of my recovery, the bottleneck of my discharge, the Goddess further challenged me with countless variations of balancing exercises. She had more moves up her sleeve than that penguin, a larger variety than a packet of Arnott's Assortments. I was shifting my weight from leg to leg, reaching for and picking up objects, and walking up and down the hospital stairwell without holding on to the rail. I even surprised myself with that one!

With my eyes shut, I stepped across various surfaces while holding items in my affected hand. I bounced a ball while skipping, jumped through hoops, juggled balls of fire, walked a tightrope.

Yeah, right!

But the exercises we did do advanced my walking technique from a drunken midnight stagger to more of a tipsy early evening stroll.

Sometimes you need to read in between the lines to get the real answer.

'Will I ever walk normally again?' I asked the Goddess.

'Umm …' She paused and looked up at the ceiling. 'Well, you'll be able to dodge obstacles.' I don't know what you think, but I'd reckon that was a no.

During a conversation with Long Arm, I said, 'When I'm better, I'm going to reward myself with a classic Triumph motorcycle, or an old vintage car. What do you think?'

'Maybe an old car,' she replied.

Again, read between the lines. There was no chance I was going to ride a motorcycle again.

The task of dressing had to be executed with a certain method, precision. As you would expect, Long Arm had it covered, *nutted out*, life skills training me for beyond the comfort of these four walls.

'I'm going to teach you how to put a T-shirt on.'

*Der, McFly. I think I can work this one out on my own.*

'Okay, extend your left arm out in front of you. With your right hand, fit the T-shirt over your left hand and through the sleeve, then pull it up to your upper arm and fit your right arm through its sleeve.'

'Hang on, I think you're going to need to write this down.'

'Then pop your head through, pull it over and down and it's on. Got it? Easy, hey!'

That all sounds straightforward enough, right? But it had to be done in that exact order, *every* single time. Every!

During my stay in this fine establishment, I'd pretty much followed all directions, played by the rules. I bent like a banana when the Goddess requested, long armed when Long Arm suggested, butt wiggled when the Grooming Guardians wanted. But I'm not really the type who likes to colour in between the lines, follow the leader. Personally, I like to experiment, test the hypothesis, draw my own conclusion. Yeah, I know ... what can I say? I live on the edge!

Mental note—*Follow Long Arm's dressing method! Every!*

Through this medical vernacular head spin, this *physiology crash course*, one of the things I learnt, amongst many, was that when there is damage in an area of the brain, other parts of the brain have the ability to rewire themselves and form new connections to compensate for the damaged area, executing tasks that the damaged part once performed. This is medically known as neuroplasticity, and over the last twenty odd years its scientific understanding has greatly evolved, replacing the century-old belief that the brain is hardwired and that damage is irreversible.

There's an interesting book by Dr. Norman Doidge called *The Brain That Changes Itself*. The book contains many stories about neuroscientists across the US conducting experimental brain therapy treatment on patients many years after their injuries occurred using the principles of neuroplasticity. Some examples of recovery achieved by these patients range from regaining the ability to walk after doctors had declared it impossible to a debilitatingly stroke-affected elderly man recouping his physical ability after his initial hospital rehabilitation therapy ended.

In many ways, neuroplasticity hasn't impacted mainstream medical practise as of yet. However, it was another reassuring benefit, along with the revelation of age, to know that recovery can occur over one's entire lifespan, not just in the two-year 'statistical' timeframe I was told—advice that acts more as a temporary safety net, a buffer zone, rather than medical fact.

Although the word 'neuroplasticity' wasn't a dominant part of the crash-course curriculum during my time in rehab, what we were practising was exactly that in its infancy.

With all of my significant improvements—when not left alone at night with a low spirit and nagging fatigue, attempting to fend off the dirty demon lurking in dark corners—I felt fiercely hopeful that I was going to be one of those success stories you hear about. I wanted to be one of those blokes who had a crazy story to tell, to be able to look back at this time with pride, honour, and dignity.

Asking for help has never been my forte. It has never come *au naturel*. Like most kids of the 'suck it up and get on with it' generation, otherwise known as those of us who grew up in the seventies and eighties, we simply had to just work stuff out for ourselves. Do what had to be done, find a way.

Handouts were never simply handed out.

Then, suddenly, I was a helpless man. A dependant person who required *help* to manage each and every little thing, and that frightened the hell out of me! Having someone wipe my backside, towel my private bits, slide my underwear on, feed me and so on did two things. One—it made me feel vastly vulnerable. And two—it pushed me to fight for my independence.

My resignation of all responsibility wasn't one I made by choice. Everyone did what needed doing to save me, to help me. The Grooming Guardians took care of all the details of daily survival needs: food, drink, hygiene. The therapists mended my body; the psych, my mind; and the doctors, my health, leaving me blown away by the care I received—*the incredible strengths of human kindness.*

All I had to do was get better, get stronger, get walking.

It was all admirably humbling being the *bystander* to my own life, watching others provide care for me. Fussing over me, making sure I was comfortable, nurturing a space for my health to be a priority. Other than when I was a child, I can't recall when I had last felt so cared for.

Discharge morning: June 25, 2009, after two months and sixteen days in hospital. In the grand scheme of life, it's not a very long time. A turtle and hare race; some days flashed by, others crawled. I was feeling unsure, uneasy, unsettled, un-, un-, un-. My independence was far better than during the assisted-behind-wiping period, but far short of the *'working it out for myself'* phase. And now, once I left the confines of this *fine establishment,* I would no longer have the luxury of relying on my rehab team to wrap me up in cotton candy.

From this day forward, till neuroplasticity further worked its magic and developed its pathways, I was going to have to make asking for help my *forte,* make it feel *au naturel.* Ask for this, ask for that; say I need assistance here, require help there. And since my rehab team weren't accompanying me to re-establish myself in the big old scary world, those helpers were going to be my family.

It became clear that Silv couldn't add any more weight to her overflowing load, her tangled ropes now trailing in the wake of self-despair—*running on empty, supplies scarce, enthusiasm low.* The 'love boat of hope' sailed without her, and I trode the deck boards alone.

I toyed with the possibility of temporarily living there, with my girls, all of us together like one big happy family. Perhaps take refuge in the spare room, bunk up with my baby girl, Maddie. But I just knew—I could feel it in my heart, felt it in my bones, and now that I was standing on the outside of the jar, the label read loud and clear. This relationship had long expired.

It left me in a scattered state, a little lost. For the past several years I'd been living at a buddy's place, but my 'independence' wasn't independent enough to return to that. I needed people's help; I had to rely on others. The idea of taking up residency at Dad's was an option, a viable one. Our old orange brick family home stood empty, as Dad lived nearby with his partner. *It'll give me some time,* I resolved.

The immediate plan was for my sister Ange to come pick me up and check me out of this cotton candy comfort—*I don't want to leave*—eject me from the warmth, the safety, the support, and inject me into the *big old scary world,* where I'd settle into Dad's. *Till I get my head straight, work stuff out.*

On the flip side of my fear, the uncertainty, were my girls. I was so looking forward to seeing them, being part of their daily lives again. No longer being a dad in hospital, their father they only visited after school—*still in uniform, homework waiting, my heart breaking*. I had missed them *so* much.

All my stuff was packed and ready to go. It amazed me the amount of junk I had accumulated whilst in rehab. I filled several bags with clothes, personal gadgets, books and magazines.

After a good going-over by the cleaners—*disinfectant lurking*—'The Hilton' would soon be ready for the next vertically challenged survivor who's nearly ready to fly the coop—*sent to the wolves.*

I made my way round the ward, limping down the halls I once was wheeled through. I dropped in on a few friendly faces to say my farewells. Snow White's parole was not up for review yet; she still had more potatoes to peel, more floors to sweep. 'Catch ya on the outside.' We exchanged numbers and made a pact to keep in touch, stay *stroke buddies.*

Back in my room, strangely savouring the last few moments before I handed my key in—*unsure, uneasy, unsettled, un-, un-, un*—I anticipated the Goddess and Long Arm popping in for a friendly visit, a last goodbye.

'Thank you so much. I couldn't have done it without you!' I wanted to cry. Again.

'Oh, I don't know. You did all the work.' The Goddess was bashful—*grinning widely like a smiley face emoji, the one with the cute rosy cheeks.* Kiwi, All-Blacks, blonde.

Long Arm still on the job, coaching me as I shoved the last of my belongings into a bag. 'Hold the bag with your left hand.' Dearly relentless—*straighten your spine, tighten those rib muscles.* I couldn't thank her enough.

Using the dressing technique that had been drummed into me, I slipped on my newly Vietnamese-tailored dark olive-green corduroy jacket, made for a quarter of the price—*look very nice, mister*—left arm first, *every*. Then I pushed my affected left leg through first, *every,* into my jeans. One of the cheery Grooming Guardians tied the laces to my favourite converse sneakers, and I was ready to rock 'n' roll.

'Hi, how are you? I heard what happened to you and wanted to tell you about my brother,' she began, her voice fragile. 'He's in the next room and had a stroke just like you.' I could feel my tears pending, building, ready to fall. 'It happened a few months ago. He's getting better, slowly, and soon he will walk again.'

She held my hand. 'Don't worry—you're going to walk again. You're going to walk out of here with my brother. We'll all walk together.'

And just like that, I walked out of hospital.

NINETEEN
# Tell Him He's Dreaming

Parading along the high street, complete with a twenty-seven-piece marching band of brass, woodwind and percussion, toe tapping, jazz swinging, punching out Queen's classic 'We Are the Champions,' the township filled with joy. There were dancing girls, pompoms, high kicks and hordes of people six deep along the curb's edge, all there to witness the spectacle, take part in the festivities. A commemorative street parade, a celebration.

Homemade banners bobbed in the air. 'Welcome Home,' they read. Council workers wearing hi-vis jackets directed us through while flashes of light from the paparazzi photographers surrounded us, eager to capture *Time* magazine's front cover shot. A Channel Seven helicopter was flying overhead as the breaking news was telecast across airwaves, onto rooftop antennas and into suburban lounge room televisions, a live bulletin interrupting midday movie.

At the end of the street stood a stage. The newly reformed Cold Chisel had just finished performing their classic 'Khe Sahn,' the last chord still resonating over the massive PA. Our slow-moving vehicle, flanked by security, was ushered to a stop by a black-dressed man. Like a celebrity arriving at a red carpet event, he opened my car door. I prepared myself for the Goddess's *shuffle, swing, brace, shift,* manoeuvre, but for the first time, I'd be going from car seat to standing position—no wheelchair.

Eager admirers, stroke groupies and more were all waiting, wanting to take a selfie with me. I happily obliged, wonky smile and cockeyed. The man in black escorted me to the stage, shepherding me through clusters of people until, with a welcoming hand, he kindly offered to help me climb the stairs. I step up onto the stage and receive a nod from Jimmy Barnes, acknowledging my achievements. The mayor greets me with a warm smile, a firm handshake. 'Welcome home, son,' he said just before he handed me an oversized pair of scissors.

Standing a few metres apart, two pretty young ladies, blondes, had a red ribbon suspended between them, their white sequined leotards sparkling in the sunlight. Stepping forward, unassisted, I cut the ribbon. Loud applause erupted, cheering, wolf whistling. 'You're a legend, Antonio!' someone shouted.

The mayor approached the microphone. With hand gestures he hushed the crowd down to a silence, made a short announcement, then presented me with the key to the city.

*Tell him he's dreaming!*

I know, I know. What can I say? I was deluded.

Of course, no such thing happened. Traffic moved as normal. People waited at bus stops and mothers pushed prams. I felt a little empty, vacant, unsure of how I was going to fit in again—*un-, un-, un-*.

We dropped into the council office and in exchange for the medical report filled out by the Mechanic, a roadworthy, they gave me a disabled badge to display on our dashboard.

At discharge, just before I left the hospital, I was loaned a wheelchair for temporary use, about a month or so. The Grooming Guardians handed it to me anticipating I would want to be wheeled out of the hospital, preserve my energy, but I wasn't having any of that. *Thanks, but I'm walking out of here—on my own two feet!*

I was only capable of short distances, as I had only walked a few loops around the hospital building with the Goddess. My endurance was still at low battery charge, not enough power for a long-distance phone call.

Awkward and peculiar, I felt like an oversized toddler, pram outgrown. Through the automatic sliding glass doors and across the large polished tiles, my sister Ange pushed me into the local plaza for a quick scoot around to grab a few essentials. Shoppers wondered and watched, conscientiously clearing a path, making room for the man in a wheelchair. It was my first real venture out in public. I'd been hoping to go unnoticed, wishing I was invisible, see-through—and whattaya know, we just so happened to bump into an old buddy.

I just wasn't ready for it; I wasn't prepared. Long Arm had somehow missed this part of 'life skills beyond these four walls' training. She mustn't have done it 'a thousand times before.'

All the un-s were suddenly pulverising, uncomfortable, uneasy, unfamiliar. I sat low in the wheelchair while he stood high in front of me. I looked up and he looked down, my one good eye trying to lock on to his good pair.

The conversation was short, staggered, full of speed humps. We made idle chitchat about nothing, this and that. I was kind of waiting for him to ask questions about my recovery, my stroke, Vietnam. *Does he even know?* I wasn't sure if he had heard. *Surely someone said something—news travels fast. What am I gonna say if he asks? How do I answer questions like 'How are you?'? It's not just a simple 'good' or 'okay'—it's complicated. At what point do I begin telling him how I am? Is it how I am right now, or how I've been lately? Do I say, 'Well, you see, I was in Vietnam and ...' or do I say, 'I'm getting better. Couldn't walk a month ago!'?*

'Yeah, man, good to see you again. Take care.' He never asked.

Wrapping my head around my own acceptance of myself was only at the beginning of this triathlon, the gunshot sound of the starter's pistol still ringing in my ears. The flipside to self-acceptance is else-acceptance—acceptance by others—and maybe the flame had been turned off, but the heat needed time to cool, simmer down into forgotten lukewarm bath water. But right now, it was still too hot for me to even dip my toe in.

Nothing had changed at all; the room looked exactly as it did some fifteen years ago. Decades-old furniture, *brown*. Missing handle on the chest of drawers, *brown*. Frosted glass lamp, *gold*. Bedside table, *brown*.

Italian retro at its finest!

Dad had emptied some of the drawers, squeezed some of the stuff he hadn't had the heart to throw out into leftover grocery bags, then jammed them into the hallway cupboard. Veneer louvered doors, *brown*, containing a multitude of childhood memorabilia.

As best I could, with 1.33333 functioning hands and Long Arm's echoing reminder—*'Use it or lose it'*—I began to unpack my hospital bags, sieve through the junk. Take stuff I had scattered around the Hilton and scatter it around my old bedroom.

The 'Use it or lose it' reminder still reverberating in my head, an echo chamber, I attempted to fold a few T-shirts and fill those now-empty drawers, give them new life, a purpose. That is, until the reality set in—that, really, T-shirt folding is a 2.0000 handed job. *Far out. I'll just shove it in there for now.*

Thanks to rehab's garment management classes, I suspended a few jackets and shirts off abandoned clothes hangers. Doable with 1.33333 hands, provided you follow Long Arm's step-by-step instructions. *Every*. She would've been proud, I thought.

Blue Tack valiantly standing the test of time, my old Jim Morrison poster was still stuck to the inside of the wardrobe Doors.

'Oh, *bello, come va*?' an old childhood friend's mum asked later on as I waddled not like Snow White, but hobbled like Charlie Chaplin down Dad's street. I made my way along the old familiar footpath, come cricket pitch, come skatepark, come whatever our youthful imagination could muster.

'*Ciao, signora, sono bene.*'

'That's a-good, my darling. Your farda tell-a me what happen. You okay?' An elderly widow now, eternally dressed in black to respect her dearly departed husband. 'You look-a good!' Her thick Italian accent was comforting.

Our orange brick family home, the base camp and call centre for diallers wanting an update, wanting info about my Vietnam battle, now had itself an old lodger—me—back again after a long hiatus.

Dad acted as my unofficial and voluntarily appointed carer. Living nearby prompted him to drop in daily, check in on his in-need son and bring food, offer transport, perform home care duties, and water his beloved-by-all veggie garden.

'*Pa, lascialo! Lo farò!*' *Dad, leave it! I'll do it!*

Like dialling in a transistor radio, searching for reception, there was a whole lot of adjusting going on. Getting used to not having cotton candy at the end of a call button meant I needed a little calibrating—*I was going to have to make asking for help my forte, make it feel au naturel.*

Normally, I was the helper, not the helpee, so it just didn't feel right—it was like fingernails across a blackboard. I'd initially struggled with it in rehab, but the wizardry of the Grooming Guardians made the reassigning of responsibility happen like magic. Plus, that's their job—they get paid for it. After an eight-hour butt-wiping, towel-jostling, salami-dangling shift, they'd go home to a pair of moccasins and a cuppa in front of the telly. But here, amongst my family, there was no escaping this.

I soon realised that I had stacks and stacks of time on my 1.33333 hands. My days were as clear as an evoking Vietnamese sky, and once I knocked out my daily morning physio routine, that clear day seemed to have no end. Other than rebuilding my life, I needed to find something to do—*fill those now-empty drawers and give them new life, a purpose.*

Now, do you remember that idea I had early on in my recovery? It was around the time that hope kicked in: *I was now going to have the most precious thing we all have so little of. Time! Time to do* the things I loved, time to do the things I wanted. One of the very first things I decided to do with my time, other than rebuild my health, was complete a music project I had been casually chipping away at for years, but I'd never had enough time. And perhaps I hadn't quite worked out how I would go about it, how I would get it done, given my present physical state. But the thrill of the idea overshadowed the hurdle of the how, and now with time on my hands—or hand—and a growing self-belief, such things were suddenly a real possibility. It's possible!

With Rem's assistance, in a spare room at dads, we assembled my basic recording equipment that'd been in storage for a number of years while I was busy doing life—*flat-out-like-a-lizard drinking*. After lots of head scratching and memory recalling, trying to get my brain-damaged brain to neuropath its way through the steps of connecting studio gear—plug in a guitar here, a microphone there, speakers, a computer—*three days later ...*

I first began by listening to recordings of the songs I wrote in between lizard living, tunes I'd bashed out on my guitar. All the recordings were pretty rough and ready, just ideas thrown together to demonstrate a song; hence where the word 'demo' came from, though you may have already known that.

So, as I sat in my makeshift simple, basic post-stroke home studio, occupying the spare room that my sisters had once shared, I listened to those songs. There were about ten of them, filled with familiar words, melodies and material. Tunes I'd composed for a bit of fun, a temporary escape from lizardry, songs I had written for no one else but myself.

But for some reason, somehow, someway, I heard these songs with fresh ears, or a fresh ear. They made my heart smile, made neurons connect, made the pain ease.

And, as simple as that is ...

I found my purpose!

Slightly elevated, gentle and soft, floating above the idle waiting room noise, just loud enough for my *kkkssshhhambled* hearing to hear: 'Antonio Iannella ... Antonio Iannella.' I looked up towards the voice.

'Hi, Antonio, I'll be your outpatient occupational therapist.' Short but Sweet smiled at me. 'Come with me.' We walked side by side, chatting—'How are you? How ya doing?'—and getting pleasantries out the way. We turned left, right, moving along familiar corridors, passing closed consulting room doors. The same corridors and closed doors I had been pushed through in a wheelchair, wearing board shorts, on my way to hydro. *Ta-ta-ta, ta, ta, ta-ta-ta, grey squirrel* routine not required—Short but Sweet had an all-access pass.

'Just in here.' She opened one of the consulting room doors and we entered, sitting at a small desk facing each other. 'So, how are you coping with it all?'

The question was clear and direct with a sincerity that instantly untangled my composure, dissolved it in a flash. *Oh, man, what's wrong with me.* I thought I had done all my crying in hospital, gotten it all out, drained my tear tank till it was tearless, dry.

'I'm sorry,' I shamefully mumbled, tears cascading like candy from a piñata.

'It's okay, don't worry. You've been through a major trauma.' I snapped Kleenex tissues out of the box at hand. 'How about I re-establish psychology sessions as part of your community rehab?'

'Yeah, okay, that would be good.' I last saw the Duke just before discharge and kinda missed the man. I needed to talk, wanted to know what the hell all my tears were about, why, when, how. *Stop.*

'Great, I'll send him an email. For now, let's make a start with some therapy.'

I had a preconceived idea that I'd be doing pretty much the same exercises I had done with Long Arm, just carrying on, but was pleasantly surprised with Short but Sweet's interpretation. So much so that I was of two minds about what to nickname her.

She placed a plastic cup, wrapped with Velcro, over towards the edge of the desk, a short reach away. 'Pick up the cup and raise it to your lips. No chicken wings!'

'What? No chicken wings?' I thought I'd misheard her—*milking the cows.*

'Yeah, no chicken wings. Ya know, keep your elbow tucked in and arm straight when you're reaching. Long arm!'

For reasons I'm not sure of, I chose 'Short but Sweet' over 'Chicken Wings' ... but I must admit, in retrospect, Chicken Wings has more comic value.

We pressed through a sixty-minute tearless OT session—bet you're proud of me, hey?—then she sent me on my way with a little goodie bag of treats. A Velcro-wrapped cup for drinking, three toy timber blocks to build a miniature Arc de Triomphe, dominos to erect Stonehenge and large handled plastic cutlery to help me shovel food.

'Find a container to store them in and leave it on your kitchen table. Use them daily. And no chicken wings!'

I soon learned the Diagram Lady (CBR physio) had a secret passion—an unpursued career, an after-hours hobby. We worked on a whole variety of physio exercises—standing, balancing, walking, reaching, bridging—that not only matched the Arnott's assortments collection of the Goddess's, but also took it one *Happy Feet* dance step further by fulfilling her artistic endeavours with neat little 2D drawings of a stick figure person demonstrating how to do the exercises. *Oh my god!* I know, right? And those drawings were always accompanied with short descriptions for those memory-affected strokers.

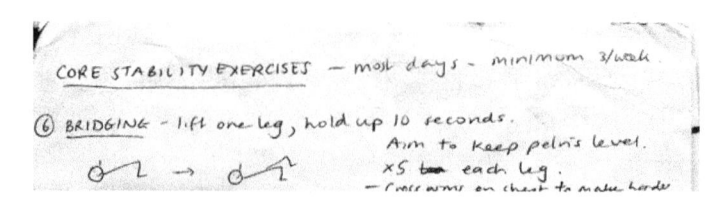

'We're going to focus on refining your mobility,' advised the Diagram Lady, 'and get you used to different environments.' Shoulder-length hair, light brown, creative, yoga. 'Indoors, outdoors, public spaces and uneven surfaces.' I was liking what I was *kkkssshhhearing*. 'We'll work on balance, walking and'—check out this last thing she said—'running.' Absolutely crazy.

Okay, so you're probably thinking, *Yeah, right, running? As if!*

It's cool, that was my first thought too. *Me, run? That won't be pretty*. Then, after giving it some careful consideration, you've probably come up with some concerns: *Hold on a sec, steady up there. Running? How is that even possible? Antonio, have you forgotten all about that spiel you bored me with about core strength? I nearly stopped reading your book, mate—it was too much! So, I must tell you, for your own sake, that running without working on core strength first isn't smart!*

Good point, and thanks for your concern. But keep your shirt on, stop stressing—the little stick figure man had it covered.

It didn't take a great mastermind to unravel the secret outpatient therapy acronym code. The list was short—PT and OT twice weekly, hydro weekly, monthly psych with the English gentleman, and a burst of speech therapy fortnightly to help iron out the last of my wonky smile.

When time permitted, in between CBR therapy sessions, I'd venture up to the rehab ward to stretch my legs, clock up some steps. Drop in on the Grooming Guardians and say a quick hello to Long Arm, the Goddess, Houdini, whoever was free and not elbow-deep in fixing broken bodies. I'd roam the rehab halls to collect kind, caring, positive comments. *Wow, look at you! Your walking is so much better. Well done!* I was in need for nurturing, something to ease my cotton candy craving.

To help me feel like I belonged.

Bystanding left me with a lot of time to burn, and a lot of that time was burnt waiting around. Waiting for this appointment, then waiting for that appointment. Waiting for someone to pick me up, and then waiting for someone to drop me off, conveniently inconvenient.

The scarcity of my independence weighed me down like a backpack full of burden. So, when the CBR receptionist kindly suggested I take advantage of the subsidized taxi service they provided, I jumped at it ... alright, maybe not *jumped,* but I did put my hand up really high. My good hand.

Once again I was waiting, waiting, waiting, *conveniently inconvenient.* Finally, my name was called. I stood and walked towards the voice.

'You've made a remarkable recovery!'

The last time I'd seen the Rowing Team's head doc was when I had just gotten back from Vietnam, all banged up and flat on my back. The Coxswain had worn me out with his soft interrogation—*follow my finger, touch my finger, pull my finger*—as the other five gender-diverse, serious-faced youngish doctors scribbled down illegible notes.

'Thanks, Doc.'

With an extended arm and open palm, he invited me into his office. 'Take a seat.'

Rolling his chair forward, lower body disappeared beneath the desk. Smart and casual dress code for patient meetings—no white coat required, stethoscopes RDO.

'I've had a good look at your scans. Your AVM is in your brainstem. With the type of surgery I perform, it's in a very dangerous and difficult location to treat.'

The neurosurgeon specialised in intrusive surgery, entering into brains to clamp whatever needed clamping, like an AVM. I know that sounds strange—it certainly did to me; it gave me a shiver—but that's how he said it, casual, toneless. He didn't go into detail. And though it's so unlike me not to ask tons of annoying questions—the Mechanic can verify—I just left it at that, totally floored.

Then he added this, flooring me even further: 'An AVM has a three percent possibility of a re-bleed per annum. That's fifteen percent over five years, thirty percent over ten.'

*Go easy on the mathematics, dude, you're scaring me!*

So, from what I understood, after I did some quick mathematical calculations in my head, leaving the AVM untreated wasn't 'statistically' recommended. Gotta love those statistics!

'However, I am unable to perform that type of surgery on you. It's too dangerous. One wrong move could kill you!'

'So, what do I do?'

'Just live your life.' The gravity of his toneless speech dissipated. 'I'll refer you to another surgeon who specializes in other forms of surgery. Maybe he could do something.'

I walked out of there feeling like *freshly laid bitumen, flat and black*. Again, there were no straight answers. Just more 'maybe's, an additional 'probably' and an extra 'could be'.

I made my way down the elevator, shoegazing, Chaplin-ing through the foyer and out the hospital doors. I decided to leave that whole conversation right there, in his office at the Royal Melbourne Hospital, and not entertain those frightening statistics. I'd forget all about researching what an AVM was, cease worrying about having brain surgery, and *just live my life*.

Ignorance is bliss.

TWENTY

# Neil Armstrong

Morning tea, a hot cuppa, and a couple of Monte Carlos. 'Girls, what are we gonna call it when we want our patient to stand with their feet a slight distance apart? Anyone, anyone?' said the head nurse. 'Yes, Jenny.'

'How about "feet shoulder width apart"?'

'Oh, Jenny, that is good. I like that one. Well done, love. Anyone else?'

'Yeah, I've got one.'

'Go for it, Christine.'

'Ummm, "feet separated".'

'Not bad, Christine, not bad at all. I'll just write them down ... feet separated, feet shoulder width apart. Now, everyone, let's have a vote. A show of hands, please. Okay, the first one is feet separated ... that's Christine, Erica and Joanne, makes three. Now feet shoulder width apart ... Jenny, Monique, Rebecca and Pauline make four. Well done, girls, 'feet shoulder width apart' it is!'

'When you're standing at the sink, make sure you're in the right position. Feet shoulder width apart!' At some point Short but Sweet paid me a home visit to run through a safety checklist, flag potential trip hazards. 'That step down from the shower's a bit dangerous. You're gonna need to get a mat so you don't slip.'

Apart from the awkward 'running into an old friend in a shopping centre when you're in a wheelchair' part of 'life skills beyond these four walls' training that Long Arm had missed, those therapists, all of them, ran a microscope over everything.

Along with her OH&S inspection, Short but Sweet, alias Chicken Wings, conducted an off-campus therapy session, supervising the Arc de Triomphe construction and overseeing the Stonehenge build right there on the kitchen table. 'No chicken wings.' She was barely over for an hour, and I reckon she said that at least seventeen times, making me question whether her nickname was the right choice.

'Feet shoulder width apart!' Smallest room in the house.

'Hey, mate, how are you? Yeah, the songs sound cool. I'd love to help you finish them.' Suddenly, I was buzzing with excitement, mind blown. All those lizardry years of flat out drinking, squeezing in escapism during life's tiny slithers of time, the gaps. Some of those songs I wrote took years to complete. I'd write a verse in between this, construct a chord progression in between that, a riff here, a bridge there.

Music had gone from being a lifeline to being sidelined.

Life as a grownup got real. Adulthood got serious. I had kids to raise, bills to pay, school runs to do and cats in the cradle. Suppressing my love for creativity, expression and passion felt all but inevitable, pushing it so far down it barely saw light, got air. I traded it all in for stability: an income, holiday pay, sick leave, dedicating myself to being a father, which I adored. But now there I was, ejected out of that life and unable to return, not wanting to return—the Severing. And maybe I'm sounding like one of those crazy blokes who's got something NQR going on in his head—we all know one!—but stroke, as horrible as it is, has awarded me with a return to my oldest love: music.

*Circulo completo.*

Now this was my opportunity, *my purpose*. I was going to grab on to it with my 1.33333 hands, hold on as tight as I could and not let go.

And just like that song John and Paul wrote for Ringo, 'With A Little Help from My Friends,' after me swallowing my pride and asking for *assistance*, surrendering to the reality that I couldn't do it on my own, my old musician buddy Machine Man—who I hadn't seen, nor heard from in a dozen years—accepted my Facebook friend request and agreed to join my campaign of purpose.

Back in the day, guitar players were aplenty. If someone chose to pick up an instrument, most likely it was a guitar. However, not many of those abundant guitarists could match the virtuosity of the well-oiled Machine Man.

Machine Man wasn't like the Mechanic; let's not mix the two up. He didn't just stand at the foot of the car with his head under the bonnet—*Can ya bring it in Chewsday?*—ah-ah, he was all over it. Before our dozen years of no contact, as aspiring young musos playing in bands together, he'd jump from guitar to keyboards, bass, then drums, and finally sing. A show-off!

An old mate used to say, 'A name doesn't make a band. It's the band that makes the name!'

Lupe Velez was a glamorous Golden Age actress. I first heard about her on that American sitcom *Frasier*. Her popularity had begun to wane, and her career hadn't quite hit the heights she'd imagined. In a final attempt to become immortalised, forever remembered, she planned this lavish suicide. Staged her bedroom with candles, flowers, silk sheets, did her hair and makeup, dressed in a pretty white nightgown. Then she swallowed a large number of pills, lay on her bed and imagined how beautiful she'd look in tomorrow's newspapers when they found her dead.

However, after eating her final meal, she began to feel queasy—bit like I did after my enema—the pills evidently not mixing well with her final enchilada combo plate. Feeling nauseous, she raced into the bathroom, tripped and fell headfirst into the toilet.

And that's how they found her!

Lupe's story was tragic, and I thought Velez would make for an interesting band name. Something that may prompt people to ask about, something quirky—*not so obvious*.

'Let's put it on the list.'

Although the fate of Miss Velez, portrayed on *Frasier*, was predominately made up of Hollywood myth and legend, her meticulously orchestrated suicide in a staged room, surrounded by flowers and candles and with immaculate hair, makeup, and nightgown, happened as planned. She was found the next morning by her secretary lying on her bed, looking glamorous, just like how she imagined.

Still sad, though.

The band names shortlisted were all as silly as each other. Molly suggested Flying Pig; Charlotte, Kangaroo History; and Maddie had nothing, still wrapping her head around saying 'Dada'.

Last up on our silly list of band names was boycriedwolf, as in the fable. And before you call the literacy police on me for not using a capital *B* on boycriedwolf, we deliberately spelt it with a lowercase *B*, as it has better symmetry that way—boycriedwolf. See?

One of the hardest things about being in a band is finding a name that everyone agrees on. Luckily, it was only me and Machine Man who had to agree, and perhaps he didn't dig the irony of Velez, as he took a shining to boycriedwolf—with a lowercase *B*.

A giant tin of beans, I was, and the Duke, a can opener, prying me open and then listening as I spilt the beans. It appeared that my tear tank had a deep supply of reserves, enough spare fuel to cry me a river. We wrestled life with stroke, hurts from love, fear, guilt, grievance, solitude, sadness. And though boycriedwolf provided a fire exit for the worst of the heat, I was still a smorgasbord of emotions.

Learning to adjust to this life outside *these four walls* was a Russian roulette wheel of how you're going to feel on any given day at any given hour, any minute. It's perhaps why Long Arm never covered it in her life skills training; it's just not possible to easily find alternative approaches to unreliable emotions.

My head would be in a spin, *time warped, thick, and heavy,* swinging from being completely immersed in the joy of making music again. Working on the songs with Machine Man and recording in my post-stroke home studio gave life new purpose, gave me something to work towards.

*Circulo completo.*

Then days, hours, or even minutes later, once the boy had exhausted his cries, out came the wolf—most likely the same one that had lurked in those dark corners of my wardroom—stalking around me menacingly before it pounced. **WHAM!**

I was shifting through a phase of personal discovery, undergoing the life skills training in real time. I was painfully uncovering what I couldn't do anymore, confronting the *dark truths* that no one can prepare you for—a disabled life, and how we take so many simple, simple, simple things for granted.

My first attempt to contend with a locked door while carrying something in my good hand flipped me like a pancake, *golden brown*. I tried to unlock the door with my dodgy hand, having to take a moment to prepare my body for the 'feet shoulder width apart' approach. Three minutes later ... I gave up, frustrated, punch-drunk. I repositioned my body again, *feet shoulder width apart,* and transferred what I was carrying into my dodgy hand, making sure I had a solid *C* grip, then unlocked and opened the door with my good hand. Finally, I stepped outside only to discover that so much time had passed, I had forgotten why I was going outside in the first place.

*Heavy-duty wash cycle.*

Duke scrutinized the ingredients to my mixed menu, stripping down the elements and offering up alternatives, suggestions. It was he who introduced me to the book *The Power of Now* that I mentioned at the beginning, through the first few pages 'The past gives us identity, the future brings us fulfilment, but we rarely live in the now.'

I had no idea of how many levels of hurt I had stacked upon each other until the elevator stopped at each floor. All those years of holding on to nothing, of holding on to a failed marriage in vain ... for all those *tumultuous years,* I'd never really dealt with the associated anguish that I carried for so long. I just pushed it aside, hoping it would disappear. Then stroke reared its ugly head, and all those undealt-with emotions came crashing down around me, exploding like a forgotten landmine.

The battle of not being part of my girls' daily lives was killing me. I hadn't expected that this time spent sorting myself out at Dad's was going to be so painful. They had rocked my world, and now my stroke had rocked theirs, *tornado torn.* The guilt was burning me up inside, and I needed the Duke to help put the fire out.

More often than not, he wouldn't say much. He'd just listen, give me space to *spill the beans.* Then, metaphorically speaking, he'd take me by the shoulders and point me in the right direction, giving me enough courage to take the next step forward—*he had my back.*

Once half full of non-alcoholic Dutch courage and equipped with an extra nudge by the Chicken Wings and Diagram lady, I was ready to keep moving, putting one wobbly foot in front of the other—*living my* 'new' *life.*

'There you go, mate, I'll let you off here.' The closest bus stop to home was a few blocks away, and as the regular bus driver noticed the frequency of my bus trips, he kindly dropped me off at the top of my street along his route.

Like having hives, an itch of independence began to surface, demanding to be scratched. My life skills needed training out in the *big old scary world*—in public, in real time. That was the only way to learn. *Head on.*

'Thanks, bud, see you next time.' While carrying a few grocery bags, occasionally eyeballing my dodgy hand to see if I hadn't dropped the milk—*spilt milk*—I'd foot pedal a few hundred meters back to base camp, saying a quick hello to the senora if she were out there standing by her yellow brick fence, checking the post, hoping to see someone, anyone.

The independence itch grew, spread. Bus trips to the local shopping precinct didn't fulfill my desire; I needed more, wanted more. Facing it *head on*, I rode the train into the city, rubbing shoulders with Melbourne's eclectic mix of commuters.

It felt like I was floating in my own orbital bubble, a secret world. There but not really part of it, disconnected, I dwindled down my spare time by watching people. Seeing them rush to meet a train, barging through queues on the escalator, standing idle on platforms, checking their phones for the time, writing text messages. *Be there soon, train's late.* All the while, I just casually made my way, with time to burn, out of the station, onto a tram and across the city. Then I'd Chaplin my way into the Royal Melbourne Hospital, go through the foyer and wall gaze up the lift, arriving early—*waiting, waiting, waiting*—for another appointment with one of the Rowing Team's neurosurgeons, only to hear, 'Sorry, I can't perform surgery on you. It's too dangerous.' Then I'd be handballed onto another surgeon. 'Someone will contact you in three or four weeks.' *Patient, patience, patient.*

The sweet taste of independence lingered like a Werther's Original, but it wasn't enough! *I wanted more! I needed more!* So, I then began pestering Short but Sweet (SBS) about getting back to driving.

The 'get back to driving' conversation went something like this.
Me: 'Hey, I want to drive again.'
SBS: 'Okay, but you're not ready to drive yet!'
Me: 'I want to drive again. And I want to drive before Christmas in a few months!'
SBS: 'Yeah, sure, but you're not ready. Maybe next year.'

Me: 'What do I have to do to get back to driving?'

SBS: 'You have to go through the VicRoads driving program ... and besides, there's an eight-week waiting list before you even get started. But you're not ready yet!'

Me: 'How about you put my name down on the list and when it's my turn, I'll have a go at it? If I fail, at least I know I'm not ready.'

**Two Weeks Later**

*Ring, ring.*

'Hello.'

'Hi, is that Antonio Iannella? I'm calling from the Driving Program Department at Sunshine Hospital. I would like to make an appointment with you for your driving test.'

As they say, it's not what you know, it's who you know!

Before I was given the all clear to tear up the bitumen, I had to provide the Driving Program Department a VicRoads medical report to be filled out by the CBR doctor I saw from time to time.

The report had to demonstrate that my NQR brain could still differentiate between left and right, red and green, stop, go, and so on. Plus, there were a whole host of other requirements: ability, understanding, cognitive function and—the one that could potentially make my Christmas driving dream come undone—sight.

'I'll measure six metres back from the eyechart, where you will stand and read out the letters.' Tall, lanky, self-assured, standing in front of the chart pinned to the physio gym wall, Neil Armstrong (CBR doctor) began pacing out the six metres, taking huge steps as though the Earth lacked gravity and he was walking across the moon. He stopped at the sixth step.

'There, that's six metres. Stand here.' He drew an imaginary line with the edge of his heel.

'Gee, six metres. That looks more like twelve to me!' I stood at the invisible line. 'Ummm ... *A*?' He could see I was squinting, scrunching up my rubbery face in a desperate attempt to narrow in my vision. All I could read was the top letter, standing there all on its lonesome above all the others, almost waving at me, trying to get my attention, from twelve meters away.

'Hmm ... your vision doesn't quite meet the standards. You'll need to see an optometrist to maybe get some glasses. And get them to fill out the vision section of your medical report.'

An appointment was made as soon as possible.

'Your brain will adjust,' said the optometrist.

'But everything is out of proportion!'

'It'll take time, but your brain will learn to see with the dominant eye. Don't worry!'

FYI—being told not to worry didn't stop me from worrying!

Since I had already been wearing contact lenses for decades, the eye doc suggested I just wear one lens in my good eye, as I had been doing since my stroke. And now with a new updated singular lens, *SLR*, that would mean I'd have decent sight from one eye, my champion left, and not-so-decent sight from one blurry eye, my disobedient, flying solo right. And according to VicRoads, one good eye is all you need to drive! *Nice.*

'It'll just take time for your brain to work out which eye to see through.' Now, I could stop worrying.

The medical report had a shortlist of rules I needed to abide by in order to one day 'Hit the Road Jack': a patch to be worn over my right eye, a vehicle with an automatic transmission, a right-sided indicator arm, and for one-handed driving, a spinning knob mounted to the steering wheel, similar to one used on a forklift— also handy for texting when driving. The driving program coordinator wasn't overly impressed with that joke!

VicRoads were gonna have to try a whole lot harder to catch this old duck on the back foot. Stroke hadn't wiped out my road rules database; with my memory unaffected, the multiple choice questionnaire was a breeze. I was now ready to burn some rubber.

Thrusting my weight forward, I yanked the driver's seat into the *nervous nanna* position, steering wheel at my chin. We went through the customary pre-driving safety checks: mirrors, seatbelt, stereo. Then, with a foot on the brake, I reached my right arm across my body to shift the automatic transmission into drive, as suggested by the driving instructor. If Long Arm were in the car, she'd probably have given birth right there on the backseat, brought on by the stress of watching me not use my affected left hand to select the gears—*Use it or lose it*. But there was too much going on all at the same time, and my NQR brain couldn't process it fast enough.

'Slowly follow the road to the exit, then put your indicator on to turn left.' I felt like I was eighteen years old again, but far less confident, nowhere near as cocky.

I'd only had one previous driving lesson the week before. Fast approaching was the Christmas rush, leaving little time to spare, and my dream of driving was on Santa's gift list.

The instructor was seated to my left, advising me on how to drive. My good ear was in direct alignment with his lips, message loud and clear, while the examiner was seated in the back, quiet.

The Tour de Sunshine rolled through suburban backstreets cocooning the hospital, unfolding into neighbourhoods. We drove down side streets, traversed roundabouts and crossed traffic lights into endless areas you would only know if you lived there.

Left, right, red, green, stop, start. Every decision was made consciously, nervously, deliberately. Unnaturally, as my autopilot was asleep. Like Vietnamese TV, driving felt foreign, consuming, confusing—*too much going on at the same time*. Maybe Short but Sweet was right. I wasn't ready!

'When it's safe, pull over to your left.' The examiner watched my every move *like a hawk*. 'Okay, you're doing well. I'll give you some advice: slow down! I want you to approach an intersection with caution. Start slowing down well before and prepare to stop.'

Now, if you're thinking I was blessed with Dad's lead foot driving gene, I can assure you I wasn't; it's more habit than genetics.

Twenty years of a driving technique is hard to break with your autopilot not really asleep, just absent-minded.

'Indicate left. Once clear, take the freeway entrance.'

Taking the examiner's advice, I casually steered the car like I was cruising the scenic route of unspoilt countryside, just nudging the vehicle forward along the freeway's on-ramp. Daydreaming of the beauty of the pastures, admiring the green rolling hills, the grazing sheep.

*Hello! Wake up!* Just as we were about to merge onto the screaming freeway, I was snapped out of my pasture-green trance of those daydreaming hills and slapped into panic mode by the thud of the driving instructor ferociously slamming down the emergency accelerator at his feet in a frantic attempt to get this teeny tiny Toyota Corolla up to the speed of the bulleting freeway traffic heavyweights.

*Beeeeep, reeeooow, beeeeep, reeeooow.* Horns, headlights, high beams flashing, blaring. The sight of green pastures instantly switched to a battleground, a life-sized *Mario Kart* game. Not like the crazy, relentless Saigon traffic seamlessly flowing together, here in Melbourne, Victoria, Australia, we had rules to our road rules.

Our teeny tiny Corolla had to muscle its way into the stream, fight for a position amongst the big boys. The fuel-efficient four-cylinder was stretched to its limits, guzzling petrol to get its lightweight body moving along.

Swamped, frozen, I was shaken by my inability to deal with the situation—*this is probably why she said I'm not ready yet*. It wasn't looking likely that I'd be nominated for the driver's Brownlow Medal.

Damn you, stroke!

Feeling crushed, disappointed—*Oh, man, I've blown it*—we continued on for twenty minutes further, using up the remaining allocated time by circling suburban roads, unknown neighbourhoods, roundabouts, traffic lights. Then we were back to the familiar and safe grounds of the hospital, through the car park that

I had eyeballed each morning through my spotless rehab room window.

I pulled the Corolla into an empty drop-off bay beside the CBR entrance and slipped the auto transmission into park.

'Okay, that was pretty good. I think after a few lessons, you'll be ready to drive.'

The last week before Christmas, businesses were winding down, shopping centres were packed with shoppers and the hospital staff wore Santa hats.

I sat in the driver's seat once again, the driving instructor to my left and examiner at my back.

'Slowly follow the road to the exit'—going back through the same steps—'then put your indicator on to turn left.' This time, not like the last, I felt far more confident, cocky. Almost eighteen again.

Turning left, I pulled out of the car park. Then I booted the red Corolla to a comfortable suburban speed—not too fast, but not at *nervous nanna* speed. The unfamiliar neighbourhood quickly became familiar, the streets, roundabouts and traffic lights recognisable.

I felt ready!

There was no dismal freeway episode. I entered and exited at the appropriate speed, flowing into the stream seamlessly without the countryside daydreaming, almost like I had done it *a thousand times before.*

After thirty minutes of the Tour de Sunshine, day two, I returned to the hospital car park, manoeuvred the car into an empty car space, slipped the transmission into park and turned to the examiner.

She was smiling.

TWENTY-ONE

# Conspiring Universe

The golden rule for my girls while I'm driving is: DO NOT DISTRACT DAD! No screaming, no shouting, no fighting and especially no calling out, *'Dad, Dad, I think I'm gonna vomit!'* Just suck it up, buttercup.

Often on journeys, they'd love to discuss the great mysteries of the universe. Unravel Galileo's discoveries, state evolutionary facts and debate creationism.

Question 1: By two-year-old Maddie

'Dad, do spiders wear shoes?'

Theory 1: By ten-year-old Charlotte (Newton)

'Dad, I have a theory about the infinity of our universe ... you see, each and every day as more people are born, when they breathe, it pushes the end of the galaxy further and further away!'

Fact 1: By seven-year-old Molly

'Uh-hmm ... Dad, did you know you can't sneeze with your eyes open?'

*'Ha-choo.'* Whattaya know, she's right.

Great convos, but nothing tops this driving game of cryptic 'I spy.'

Maddie, age four: 'I spy with my little eye ... something beginning with *R*.'

'Radio?'

'No.'

'Road?'
'No.'
'Roof?'
'No.'
'... Oh, we give up.'
Maddie's answer: 'Wrapper.'
They rock my world!

We're on a mission from God—*The Blues Brothers*.

Six months of charging like a Pamplona bull saw the completion of boycriedwolf's debut album. With some nifty editing to my pre-stroke recordings, I was able to salvage a huge chunk of what was already there before my six-string heartache blanketed my musical ability, and with Machine Man's virtuosity, he effortlessly jumped from one instrument to another, recorded all the vocals and added bits and pieces, bringing my dream closer to reality.

The earliest conception of this idea—to make an album—began somewhere in 2003, shortly after the folding of Urshabloom, our London indie band I co-created. However, it had been interrupted by my return back to Melbourne—*minus a music career, but with a suitcase full of construction knowledge.*

Life doing lizardry, adulthood, and all the other cats in the cradle meant long, un-progressive intervals were part of the repertoire. Though at times frustrating, the tiny slithers of music-making time, *escapism*, mixed with long dormant gaps of nothingness provided a perfect name for the album: *intervals*.

This time with a lowercase *I*.

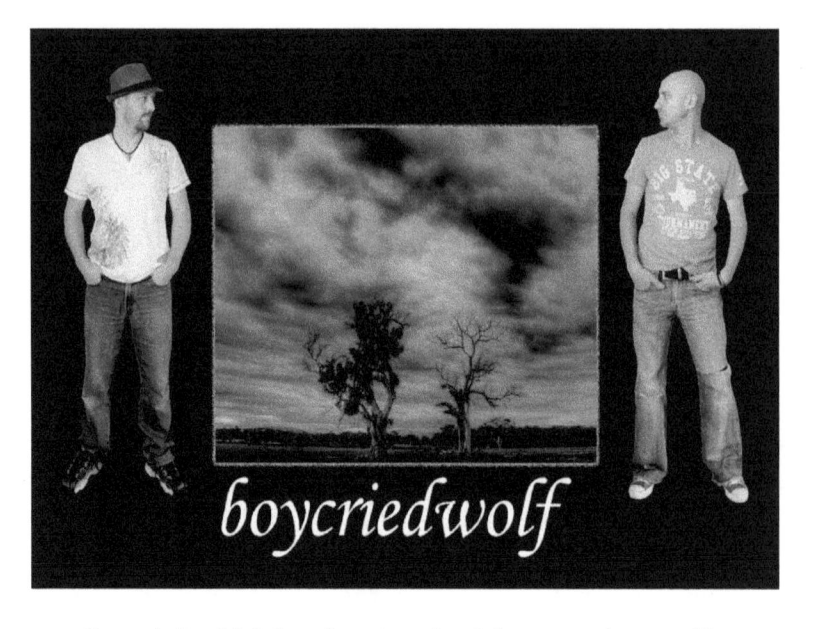

(boycriedwolf: *left*- Adam Roach, *right*- Antonio Iannella. Design and photography by Darren Roach)

A mate with a camera and some crafty design skills put together our artwork, a short run of CDs were pressed—remember, this was 2010; people still listened to CDs back then—and our mission was accomplished.

'Well done, bud, we did it! Thanks heaps, dude.' I was content to leave it at that, happy and fulfilled to have finally finished the songs and put them to bed. This little long-running, mostly dormant project had given me a purpose, something to focus on other than my health and help me *live my new life*.

Therapy for my soul.

Regardless of whether the songs were any good or not, or if the basic recording equipment met any commercial standards, all that didn't matter. I didn't care, because what those songs gave me—how I felt when Machine Man and I were recording, workshopping ideas and making music—transcended me, us, to another place, a place where the stroke demon was denied entry.

BCW, an acronym for boycriedwolf with all capitals because it has better symmetry that way—bcw ... see?—didn't have a marketing plan. So, we decided to go the organic root, old-skool. Which really means family and friends, including grandmothers.

This is the bit I love.

Without an official release and with no sales strategy, BCW began to shift a few CDs via word of mouth under the counter, a bit like that Vietnamese Motorola flip phone dude.

Our newly created Facebook page, the one and only marketing tool we had, began to attract followers. *Hey, I just bought your CD. Love the songs*! A few random messages got us all excited.

'Next up, a track called "Disconnected" by local Melbourne band boycriedwolf.' The joy of sitting in my stationary car listening to the local community radio broadcaster introduce us to the public, to the world—even if it was perhaps only a handful of local listeners tuning in—gave me such a thrill, a buzz. Having our track transmitted across airwaves, bouncing out of speakers, potentially available for anyone and everyone to hear, given what I'd been through to get to this point, was quite possibly the very first time that I truly believed that things weren't falling apart, that they were falling together. This tragedy had a reason.

*'When you want something, the whole universe conspires to make it happen.'*
—Paulo Coelho

**The Blues Brothers Restaurant Scene**
Jake: 'We're putting the band back together.'
Maître d': 'Forget it, no way!'
Elwood: 'We're on a mission from God!'

The organic buzz became the fertilizer that germinated boycriedwolf to sprout some roots and become five. *'Hey, mate, I'm putting a band together. You interested?'* The three main criteria for band member selections were: 1) nickname possibilities, 2) instrument they played, and 3) musical ability.

Machine Man had lead vocals and lead guitar covered, while impressively keeping it steady on rhythm guitar and backing vocals was his fourteen-year-old musical prodigy daughter. Young and talented—*fourteen! Wild, hey!*

When not teaching seven-year-olds how to crack someone's skull open with a single swift karate chop, Round House to the Head, a fourth dan Taekwondo instructor, also played bass guitar, covering BCW's melodic low-end groove. And last up to complete the quintet, bashing the skins and keeping time, was the handsome Italian Stallion.

As for me, I was given light duties: empty the bins and make tea, sweep and lock up after everyone's gone home ... oh yeah, and try to write some new songs. Some consideration was made to potentially play simple one-handed keyboard, but my brain was still trying to decode listening to music—*Mamma Mia*—so the thought of playing in a band with a live drummer, especially one who had guns like Arnie and hit those skins like Balboa boxing carcasses, sent my brain into *time-warped* mode, *fast and furious.*

BCW, now five strong—four for live performing, and one on light duties—began rehearsing, punching my once-dormant tunes into life. Existence.

*One small step for man, and young woman, one giant leap for man/young woman/humankind.*


'Oh, man, I'm so excited, I could just cry. After everything that's happened, I can't believe where my life's at!'

'Bud, you should be proud of yourself! Look how far you've come; you've been through so much. The CD looks cool, the songs sound awesome and the band will kill it tonight.' My brother Rem was there, supportive, out on a midweek winter's evening to witness boycriedwolf's *intervals* CD launch, our very first gig.

*One, two, three, four.* From the very first count in, the songs bounced off the stage with a charged energy, a purpose that, for me, put the icing on the cake of this whole journey. And maybe only a handful of punters knew the whole story—*Vietnam, stroke, recovery*—but that charged energy, that sense of purpose made my heart swell.

I may sound a little modest here, though I'm biased, my description likely blinded by my affection for boycriedwolf. The band just shone on stage; the songs glistened so brightly, it was like staring right into the sun.

A first-time experience for me: listening to my own songs, written from a place deep down inside, from my soul, and now, after everything, being performed by others—*a bystander*. Words, lyrics, melodies, self-confessions and three-minute-long memoirs set to music, to a beat, framing a time when my life was heading in new directions. Leaving London, quitting Urshabloom, ending a lifelong dream.

The songs were my secret little treasures, Charlotte, Molly and Maddie's siblings. Family. They brought me back to that place I most loved to be, lost in music. Back to me, to my heart. Providing escapism in between lizardry, even if it was for a short while—a quick hit, just enough air to carry on with the things we do in life that really, let's face it, are just a means to an end.

Up there on the stage, watching and listening to the fab four perform was surreal, doing it because they love music just as much as I do, but also because there was a greater purpose, a reason: to help their little lackey friend fulfill a dream.

Whether this gig was gonna be a one-off occurrence or BCW were going to keep charging forward like that Pamplona bull, it *didn't matter. I didn't care,* because right there in that moment, on a cold midweek winter's evening somewhere in the middle of Melbourne, I felt a warmth that not even stroke could chill.

Reading notes from my medical file, designer framed glasses perched at the end of his nose, the oncologist tried to convince me that microwaving my brain with radiation would be the best way to treat my AVM.

His impressive, neatly ironed slacks and cool Italian leather boots just weren't enough to win me over. As usual, I needed more information, more details, before Radioman here was granted clearance to repeatedly quick cook my brain.

I had questions.

These are the answers I received:

1. I may experience a five percent loss to the recovery I had already made.

2. I may experience headaches for a short while during and after the treatment.

And my favourite answer—not a *good* favourite, more of a WTF moment:

3. My head would be bolted to a bed beneath the radiation machine to prevent me from moving during the procedure.

Then Radioman continued to explain the process, elaborate. 'A series of radioactive laser beams will beam into your brain at a precise location. The laser beams fuse right at the point of your AVM and obliterate it.'

Obliterate! Of all the words he could have used to describe treatment, he chose 'obliterate'. I mean, he could have said 'heal,' 'fix'—even 'terminate' would have been okay—but just not *obliterate*! It sounded more like he was commissioning the US Army to conduct air attacks on a small village in Afghanistan in an attempt to flush out the Taliban.

'Have a think about it. We'll get you back in for another chat, answer any questions you may have.'

'It'll be good for you to live on your own again,' encouraged Short but Sweet. 'Doing everything for yourself will help with your recovery.'

I was nearing forty; I didn't want to live under Dad's roof forever. *Time to take this new life another step forward, complete my need for independence.*

'Yeah, great, but how will you manage on your own?' My sister's eyebrows were raised.

Life had sent me on a wild new adventure. It had thrown some massive challenges at me, and hey, I was still standing, so living back out on my own made me feel like I was doing it for the very first time. Excited.

During my hospital stay, when I began to set goals and make myself promises, I vowed, with muted tears and the love for my mum burning in my heart, to take the best of my old life and rebuild it into a new one. A reboot.

And this opportunity to go out into *the big old scary world* and live independently, to face it *head on,* was something I had to do. Something I *must* do to prove to myself that I wouldn't allow the dirty demon that stroke is to dictate my life.

'I'll find a way, Ange!'

Although my therapy appointments had been downgraded to one day a week, the approach to treatment was definitely upgraded. The Diagram Lady had me skipping, hopping, leaping, and you know how I told you she planned to get me running? *Me, run? Yeah right*. Well, she did it—sort of. I don't know if you could really call it 'running,' per se ... if you were to imagine how the lovechild of C-3PO from *Star Wars* and Charlie Chaplin would run, then that would give you a pretty good idea of my technique.

It wasn't pretty!

'So, it's been cold lately hey?' SBS tried to distract me with idle conversation. 'Just down here,' she said as we circled the rehab corridors. I held a pint of sugar in my affected hand, testing my ability to do two things at the same time: walk and carry. I don't think she was aware of my caveman theory—*Caveman's Mate: Dude, you can totally do those two things at the same time. Caveman: Shhh!*—but I just went along with it. I didn't want to be the one who ruined this 2.5-million-year-old cushy ride for us men.

'I'm going to hold your right arm behind your back.' My wrist was soon wrapped in by SBS's small hands, arm pinned behind me, a citizen's arrest. 'And I want you to hang those clothes on the clothesline with your other arm.' I wondered if the clothes were hers from home. Perhaps she was taking advantage of my good nature and getting me to hang her laundry. 'No chicken wings!'

I drove myself to my weekly CBR therapy appointments from my new digs. It was the cherry on top, liberating not only for me, but for Dad, too. His superstar self-appointed carer position now relinquished, he could return to his leisurely golden years lifestyle, food harvesting and moonshine making. *Saluti*.

'Statistically'—you know how I love statistics—'one in three people experience depression during the five years after their stroke.' Neil Armstrong's voice was doctorial. 'It's common for stroke survivors to feel this way.'

It just didn't make sense; it confused me like a lost tourist in a big city. I had so many positives going on in my new life: boycried-wolf, my own place, getting to see my girls, friends and family. Yet there I was, dealing with a darkness that only came out at night—*late lonely evenings were when the desolate wolves came beating at my door.*

Psych sessions with the Duke had wound down to make room for new patients needing emotional rescue. I was kind of okay with that, thinking I had a handle on my internal affairs.

Wrong!

As time prevailed, the boiling bath water of self-acceptance was still too hot for me to comfortably bathe in, the plug on my psychology sessions pulled far too early.

Twelve months into my recovery, I faced surprising discomfort. It was spontaneously brought to my attention when, in the company of a group of strangers, talking about the moment Vince Vaughn gate-crashed my life without a monsoon rainfall of tears was near impossible.

Whilst in rehab, hours, days, weeks after Mr. Vaughn's unannounced arrival, once my rubber-band lips were able to almost form words, I had told everyone and anyone. Whoever was prepared to listen had heard me filter through my stumbling, mumbling description of how my life had unravelled like *spindle on a spool*.

It had been far easier then, during the earlier stages of my recovery, to talk about that day. Easier to relive those last few moments, just before I got on my hands and knees to crawl through those elaborate war tunnels, than it was now, a year later.

Granted, there had still been still buckets of tears, *enough to cry me a river,* but they were different tears. They had fallen faster, felt lighter than the tears I shed now. Back then I had cried and cried and cried, in fear, in shock, in pain. But now I cried spontaneously in grief—without warning, hitting em hard and heavy, like a one in one-hundred-year storm.

As soon as I nudged anywhere near that moment—*We were about to enter underground war tunnels*—that would be my trigger, chucking it down, snot and all.

Clearly, I was still carrying the trauma.

My brain-damaged brain was too naïve to understand it, not skilled enough to accept it. I had no real knowledge of depression's muscle, of its power. I had always been an upbeat person, saw the glass half full.

And though it wasn't so long ago that Dr. Armstrong had tried to enlighten me with depression- and stroke-associated statistics, back then in 2010 when I carried the monkey on my back, mainstream discussions about the black dog weren't part of everyday vocab like it is these days. It just wasn't openly spoken about.

I was in denial.

'Is life still worth living?' Probing, as if inspecting the moon. 'Do you have thoughts of inflicting self-harm?' Neil's tone was unfaltering.

'No, not really.' I paused, thinking, feeling. 'Sometimes I wish I had just died on that day rather than having to go through all this.'

'Hmmm ... I think you really need to seek some help. Maybe consider more counselling, or perhaps medication! Have you got a regular GP?'

I'd never really had a GP that I saw regularly. I'd had no need; I hardly ever got sick. Through my search, I discovered that a decent doctor is a bit like a trustworthy mechanic: hard to find. *Greasy smile, dirty cloth, head under bonnet.*

'According to this checklist, you have depression,' said my new doc, an ex-pilot turned general practitioner. 'We can treat it with antidepressants or counselling.' So, as you can imagine, inventing a nickname for the ex-pilot came easy.

The depression diagnosis was a bit like organising your own surprise party, but the strange thing was, I was still surprised. Or, to be more precise, *in denial.*

This stroke learning curve, the *physiology thrash course* that I had been involuntary thrust into, seemed to have no end. There were chapters upon chapters upon chapters of unexplored challenges that had to be read, felt, experienced.

Just as I was reconstructing my new life, beginning to live it, I was confronted with yet another obstacle to climb. The trauma had such deep ruts that no preparation could sidestep the pitfalls; no amount of cotton candy could soften the blows.

It was around this time I coined the phrase 'The only thing predictable about stroke is, it's unpredictable!' That's how I felt. Each day was different—every morning, afternoon, and evening I was susceptible to whatever the hell depression wanted to do with me that day, vulnerable to wherever stroke wanted to take me.

Some nights it would send me on a wild ride through anxiety, a crazy trip of panic vicing my chest, constricting my lungs. Pinned down by an invisible weight, air was drawn forcefully through as I attempted to siphon oxygen, desperate to breathe deeper, slower, calmer. By midnight, a few hours later, the physical stress would cause my stroke-affected left side to throb with intense pain, *like a million tiny jackhammers penetrating my skin. Cling-filmed face, rubber-band lips.*

Then, when I should have been sleeping in the wee hours of the morning, it would finally let go, let me fall into depths I'd never been to before. So low, so deep, so dark, there was no light. And just when I'd feel I wanted it to all end—*'Sometimes I wish I had just died on that day rather than having to go through all this'*—the lights would turn on. I could breathe again. I had hope.

'I don't want to take medication to deal with this, doc.' I was hell-bent on the 'organic' thing. 'I've always been a positive person.' Other than the general stigma that came with antidepressants, my apprehension had no real grounds of reason. 'I'd prefer to try counselling first,' I concluded, adamant to fight this without chemical intervention.

Keep it *au naturel.*

Now, it seemed that the medical professionals overseeing my health had all effectively, at some point, piloted large vehicles of transport. Neil Armstrong, Apollo 11 and the Pilot had all commanded commercial aircrafts. So, it felt right—*meant to be*—to name my new counsellor Captain for her remarkable ability to steer my lost-at-sea emotional sailboat back to the shore. Dry land.

All those levels of hurt that I had visited with the Duke still required more exploring. Much of it was building rubble, decaying foundations, collapsing walls, and with the Captain's guidance, we began sorting through what was worth salvaging.

I'd say it was around this time, when the lights were temporarily on, that I began to grasp the true nature of what recovery actually meant—well, what it meant for *me,* at least. The physical component that receives most of the limelight is often the standard by which we measure the quality of our recovery.

However, what was beginning to rise to the surface, *snot and all,* was how the road to emotional recovery far extended beyond the physical. It spanned leagues ahead, and perhaps this is the reason for the statistic *'one in three people experience depression at some point during the five years after their stroke'*. In my eyes—or eye—through my experience, which was still unfolding, I needed more focus on that wrinkly walnut of a brain that was responsible for our thoughts and feelings. That squishy little nugget needed to share more of the stage.

'When you feel the anxiety begin, stop what you're doing and take a few moments to breathe deeply.' The captain stood confidently at the helm, her advice simple, common sense. 'Close your eyes and take a deep breath through your nose.' I'd never experienced anxiety like that before. I just wasn't myself; I felt out of control. 'Fill your belly with air, hold it for five seconds, then slowly exhale through your mouth.'

Last Band Standing—thirty-five bands, five heats and six thousand dollars in prize money.

boycriedwolf took to the stage fourth up on the bill of six bands. They didn't waste any time, slamming through a stellar seven-song set in a cool fashion that oozed charm. Rewarded by being named the runners-up in this lucrative Melbourne battle of the bands catapulted us into the next round.

Feeling so exhilarated, so high, was an instant lift out of the depths of depression, inspiring me to try write some new songs. By default, the piano was going to be my instrument of choice, but to say I played like a one-armed Billy Joel would have as much truth in it as this well-known presidential admission: 'I did not have sexual relations with that woman.' However, it was a work in progress.

Float like a butterfly, sting like a bee. Just like Muhammad Ali, boycriedwolf skipped through the next few heats as winners, securing a spot in the final.

*Charging like a Pamplona bull!*

The night of the grand finale, an ocean of people filled the large room. Seas of bodies gathered together before the stage as the lights blurred, heat rose, energy vibrated. I stood amongst the audience, absorbing the ambience, soaking up the excitement.

boycriedwolf opened up with the slamming 'So Surprised'. The song transformed from my initial slippery acoustic version into BCW's heavy and direct, uncompromising attack. Every snare hit, each distorted guitar strike and pounding bass line seemed to amplify the past year's events.

A few songs into the set, Machine Man hammered out the opening chords to what had become the crowd pleaser: 'Chinese Burn'.

*'Sometimes you're the one and only, sometimes you can be so lonely, sometimes you make me feel so underground.'*

'Louder, I can't hear you!' he boomed, hand cupped behind his ear.

I was in complete awe, *Sung Sot,* amongst the audience, taking it all in. Feeling the love, surrounded by swaying bodies, moving lips singing *my* lyrics, *my* words, *my* songs—it nearly brought me to tears.

It was just brilliant.

Applause eased into a gentle stir, settling for the next track.

'Here's a new one.'

'Hold Onto Me,' my first attempt at song writing since Vaughn's invasion, lyrically summed up where my head space had been lately. BCW had just learnt it at their last rehearsal, so there was a good chance it could've sounded like a bent banana, half standing. But sometimes uncertainty can produce a pearler.

The Italian Stallion counted everyone in on his sticks. The mid-tempo rhythm chugged along; it sounded tight, together, tremendous. The first verse drops in—*'I'm failing now, it's clear somehow, time has no remedy'*—and I've got tears in my eyes, my heart thumping harder than the Stallion's kick drum. *'No trust in me, my enemy, lost in the atmosphere.'* My depression nowhere to be seen, anxiety crushed by the evoking melody. *'Now I'm crawling down this lonely trail, calling out again and again.'*

My love for boycriedwolf is definitely blinding; the song sounded sublime, spectacular. The words, the music, the passion tumbling out of those speakers sent me reeling. *'Hold onto me,'* the chorus arrives, *'it's all that I need, with every breath I fear I'll disappear,'* colliding gently into the audience. Filling hearts.

*It was just brilliant.*

Copping a bashing was my hearing. Six eclectic bands—metal, rock, pop, dance—all at full throttle, smashing it out. It was a long night, with my energy running on high-octane adrenalin.

Afterwards, the judge took to the stage. 'I'm going to get straight to it and announce the winner,' she began, lips poised at the microphone.

Gathered before her, creating a passive mosh pit, bands, fans, followers, friends and family, including grandmothers, all stood waiting, hoping.

The room fell almost silent.

'The winner of Last Band Standing is …'

TWENTY-TWO

# D-Day

Defying gravity, I leaped into the arms of Round House to the Head, my chin buried in his neck, legs wrapped around his waist. Like I was a tiny two-year-old, he raised me high above the audience, gazing into my eyes like a proud father.

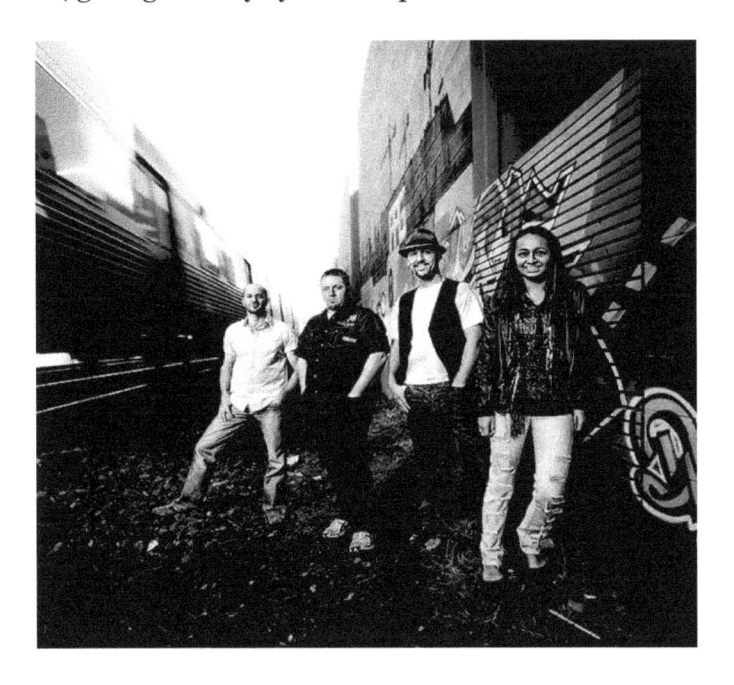

(boycriedwolf; *L-R:* The Italian Stallion, Round House to the Head, Machine Man, Young and Talented - Photograph by Simone Byrne)

Back and forth, round and round, inside out. *I could lose five percent of the recovery I've made.* I didn't know what to do, which way to go. *An AVM has a three percent possibility of a re-bleed per annum*—flooring statistics! I must admit, I was becoming a bit annoyed with doctors casually dropping stats as if my life was a cricket match—ninety-nine runs off forty-seven balls, *fifteen percent over five years, thirty over ten.* Not helpful! I was feeling trapped—damned if I do, damned if I don't.

'Live your life,' said the Coxswain. 'Clamping your AVM is too dangerous. One wrong move and …' But how do you carry on living with those odds stacked against you? The concept of 'ignorance is bliss' falls apart when you're no longer ignorant.

Silencing my better judgment, I buckled my hope to the impressive batting average of my AVM and gave Radioman clearance to commence obliteration.

What would you do?

While boycriedwolf were still howling at the moon with delight, I made my way to see Radioman to have my questions answered, accumulate more stats and, with hesitation, sign wavering consent forms with tiny printed disclaimers—<sub>we take no responsibility for any adverse effects.</sub>

'The treatment will be administered over eleven sessions in a two-week period.' We sat in a large meeting room, both of us on one side of the twelve-seater table, chairs turned slightly to face each other. 'But first we need to perform another angiogram.'

*Noooooo!* I was ready to *leg it, leg it, leg it* out of there, and this time I was able.

Still not pretty, though.

'Also, before you leave today, we'll need to make the face mask. It'll prevent you from moving during the procedure.'

The air attacks were calculated with pinpoint accuracy, radiation fusing at an exact location. If I were to flinch or move, innocent civilians could be wiped out.

'Come with me.' Radioman led me to another room, a forgotten space where top-secret medical experiments were conducted somewhere in the back of the hospital.

'Here, sit up on the table.' He stood beside me, a square bone-coloured plastic sheet in his hands. 'I'm going to heat this therma-sheet to make your mask. Lay down on your back with your head at this end.'

I swung my legs over and uneasily manoeuvred myself to lay flat, my head nestled in the saddle at the end of the table. The room was quiet, sterile, still. We were hidden in the deep confines of a large hospital, a building filled with patients, nurses, doctors and staff on other floors, on the other sides of the walls all around us, busy caring for the unwell. And though we were effectively surrounded by people, I felt so alone, empty. Just Radioman, his assistant and me, lying on my back, blankly staring at the ceiling.

In a deep stainless steel sink, they bathed the sheet in shallow warm water. After a few minutes, once the plastic softened, it was ready for use. 'Hold still.' With the help of the assistant, each of them standing either side of my head, they stretched the sheet over my face. It felt like squeezing a hand into a latex glove, the two of them fastening it to the clamps fixed to the table just beside my ears. Then with the tips of their fingers, they began moulding the mask to fit the contours of my face, kneading it around my cheekbones, chin and nose so it fit exactly. Snug.

I kept still, silent, *floored* by yet another chapter to this forever unfolding stroke journey. 'Try not to move. We just need the mask to set.' It was like being smothered with a pillow. My body was free to move but my head was locked to the table, disconcerting, the facemask's perforated holes only allowing enough air to breathe. 'Okay, keep still while we remove the mask, then you can step down off the table.' *Neatly ironed slacks, Italian leather boots.*

At last, we were ready to go, with the head clamp made, paperwork signed, angiogram booked and deployment scheduled. 'See you next week ...'

## D-Day I

I felt like I had just stepped into the future, the large modern medical machine engulfing the space, a padded table protruding beneath. The room was lifeless, strategically decorated with one motive in mind: dispensing radiation. 'You can use that chair over there to remove your shoes and jacket.' The atmosphere resembled the décor—sombre. 'Then lay on the table.'

'I'm gonna wear my boycriedwolf T-shirt to all the sessions,' I declared, *butterflies dancing*. 'The wolf will protect me!'

My fear was clear, crushing. The technician offered empathy. 'You can wear whatever you like, love'—words I needed to hear, care I needed to feel. 'Now lie down in a comfortable position. I'm going to fit the mask and screw it down to the table.' The mask closed in and cradled my face like a hammock, the darkness fractured by bits of light streaming in through the tiny air holes. She screwed my head to the table, *disconcerting*.

'I'll give you this little device to hold in your hand.' I nervously wrapped my fingers around the emergency call button, palms sweaty, thumb on the trigger. 'During the procedure, if you feel odd, just press the button.' Shockingly, I was already feeling odd. 'Try to keep still.' She left the room and made her way into the control booth, the cockpit, safely concealed behind six-inch concrete walls, protected from radiation spillage.

It was just me, all alone, *Pat Malone*. Panic button, fractured light, the future. I lay tense, stiff, riddled with cortisol. Their choice of background music was revolting, 'Lady in Red' offering no comfort.

Like a creeping missile, the radiation machine moved into position, cocooning my head, preparing itself for minuscule accuracy, precision. Awaiting the signal to release the bombs, to send radiation deep into my brain, fuse at an exact location and obliterate the enemy.

Head clamped to the bed, darkness behind the mask, Chris De Burgh romantically singing. I was cacking myself.

The stealth-like machine was totally silent, sophisticated, its target vulnerable. I wasn't sure when it was supposed to begin—would there be a signal? A countdown? What was gonna happen? Would I feel any pain?

Rigid, afraid to move, all those questions raced, worried and bounced around in my head with the radiation. It was all so quiet, too quiet. *Has it started yet?* All I could hear was the sweet lullaby about a lady dressed in red.

Thirty minutes later, the technician re-entered the room.

'All done. How do you feel?' She released my head from the clutches of the table, light returning. 'You can get dressed now.'

I sat up, swung my legs to my left, placed my feet on the floor, stood and took a deep breath of relief. The cortisol racing through my body recoiled, my heart rate eased. I felt normal.

In the corner chair I sat and dressed, then I walked down the short passage through the doors and into the waiting room where Radioman casually sat, cross-legged.

'How do you feel?'

'Not too bad, considering I just had my brain microwaved!'

'Good, you'll need to see the nurse for a minute. See you tomorrow.'

I followed the nurse into a small patient room and took a seat. 'Take these,' she said, handing me a tiny paper cup. 'They're steroid pills to help with the swelling that radiation causes. Here, drink some water.' I took a sip and swallowed the pills. 'So, what happened to you?'

I burst into tears.

Once my composure returned, I Chaplined my way out of the Oncology Department into the car park and sat quietly in my car.

I needed a little downtime to put all the pieces together, a *thinking siesta*. Talk myself into believing everything would be okay—*it's the right thing to do*. Muscle through all the barriers stroke randomly places before you, navigate the trip hazards, and find the energy, the confidence, the concentration to steer my little automatic car, with a spinning knob and a patch over my right eye, through Melbourne's shining inner-city streets all the way back to my new digs.

So, if you're wondering why I drove myself to my treatment sessions, well, you're not alone; I wondered, too. In reflection, other than me being on an independence bender and partly still grappling with asking for *help*, I was adamant not to allow the demon to dictate my life. But I'd say the main reason I transported myself in my trusty little car, like a scotty who's got no friends, was influenced by this: 'He would come in for his radiation session during a break at work and, after treatment, return to work,' advised Radioman, like it was no big deal. He had encouraged me to function 'as per normal,' and to me, driving, though harder, had become fairly normal. Many of the examples he spoke about of treatment successfully administered to other patients was what got me over the line.

I had put my trust in Radioman.

### D-Day II

I wore my boycriedwolf T-shirt again, two days in a row. I didn't care; the wolf was my guardian, my protector. The second course of treatment was a synch. My palms didn't sweat, my cortisol remained low. The future was on my side. I felt safe, relaxed—*it's the right thing to do*—fully confident in the faith of Radioman's knowledge.

My life was in his hands.

Then back through the same steps as yesterday. 'All done! You can get dressed now.' I followed the nurse into the patient room for my steroid pills, took a sip of water, swallowed and then I was back out in the car park, quietly sitting in my car, having a moment of downtime before I '*Hit the Road Jack.*'

But this time, as I made my way through the inner-city streets, Melbourne didn't shine. The tall buildings that lined St. Kilda Road were closing in on me, the trams, cars, traffic lights and pedestrians suffocating. My perception partial, I sat heavy in the car seat, my arms feeling like stone.

I spent that evening curled up on the couch, wanting to vanish. My girls were with me, so I wasn't alone, but all I wanted was solitude. *World, swallow me whole.*

D-Day III was on Monday, so I had the weekend to, as Radioman said, *function as per normal.* But that was just not possible; I felt like the top of my head was going to explode. The intensity of the headaches he had luke-warned me about drove my cortisol levels to a boiling point. My stonelike driving arms became heavy wet cement; my legs, bricks; and my balance, hearing and vision, *kkkssshhhaaammmbbblleeesss.*

Dinner uneaten, left to go cold, as the ambulance reversed up my driveway, a bright spotlight mounted to its roof flooding our front porch. With his pen torch, the paramedic gazed into my eyes— *Here we go again*—checking my vitals, blood pressure, blood sugar, heart rate. Then a casual cruise to Royal Melbourne Hospital, with no siren, in the same orderly manner as the tarmac-to-emergency chauffer ride.

Entering the hospital, beyond emergency, came with the standard scrutiny as the first time round. Stroke did not grant me instant access; the emergency doctor conducted protocols similar to a nightclub bouncer. A soft interrogation, squeezing, pinpricks, follow the finger—*the Purana Files*.

On this occasion, my head wasn't in the clouds. I had function— I could speak, sit up, stand—but everything was accompanied with a hell of a lot of pain and a sore brain wanting to spew radiation, erupt like a volcano.

Other than the physical discomfort measuring *9.5 on the Richter scale* and my anxiety, *pumping like a subwoofer,* according to the doctors, I wasn't showing a great need for urgent care. 'Once an opening becomes available, we'll get you in for an MRI.' And so I was left in a small room in emergency for several hours, periodically checked on by the Grooming Guardians.

'There doesn't seem to be any further damage.' After my MRI, I was allocated a bed somewhere up on the third or fourth floor, somewhere with city views.

The Coxswain visited me in the morning. 'The MRI shows no change to your brain.'

'But doc, I feel like death!' I spent about five days in hospital, mainly resting, trying to feel human again.

'Perhaps it was just a bad reaction to the radiation.' Other than statistics, it appeared that doctors also loved giving vague answers—*perhaps, maybe, we can't be certain.*

During my stay at RMH, I attempted to call Radioman. I needed some explanation, some reasoning, some help to process this. *My life was in his hands.* 'Sorry, he's not available. He's on holiday,' said his assistant with as much colour as the radiation room.

My volcano-like brain, accompanied by my now-boiling blood, was ready to erupt. *Away on the holiday?! What the ... ?* I had put my faith in him, trusted his judgment, relied on his support—*left in a car park, abandoned, gold coin not returned.*

After that, I pulled the pin on any further treatment!

There was no official boycriedwolf breakup; it just dissolved like a keg of Palmolive Gold.

Much to the band's surprise, too, and shortly after BCW spent their Last Band Standing fortunes on funding a full-length professional studio album that we named *distractions*—yes, with a lowercase *D*, because it looks ... grammatically wrong. The title was inspired by day-to-day life being the 'distraction': work, studying, brain microwaving—my brain, incidentally, was still cooling off—and so on, leaving my energy levels *drained like* a *day-worn battery without a charge,* which only granted me limited time in the studio. *Function as per normal ...* damn you, Radioman!

So, as I was saying, boycriedwolf's surprising Palmolive Gold fadeaway stemmed from the Italian Stallion handing in his resignation.

*How could he? This is my only chance to make something of myself!*

My disappointment with Radioman vanished. He was gone to me, and instead, all my frustration was redirected towards the Stallion. boycriedwolf had become my everything, and now my everything was quickly turning to nothing.

The whole *purpose* thing, *circulo completo,* had just lost its *purpose*. And though BCW—once two, then five, now four—was fairly confident that replacing the band's backbone was gonna happen without much effort—*'We've just recorded an album, won the band comp ... drummers are gonna be queuing to join us!'*—that mindset didn't exactly pan out organically. And so over the following days, weeks, months, our once-charging Pamplona bull lost its fight.

Feeling rather annoyed, agitated, trying to accept that boycriedwolf was pretty much over, whittled down to a paper-thin slither of soap, I stood at the kitchen sink, *feet shoulder width apart,* mindlessly doing the dishes. 'Long arm, long arm, long arm ... no chicken wings, no chicken wings, no chicken wings.'

Left hand holding a plate—'Use it or lose it'—and right hand scrubbing, I stood there thinking, drifting, scrubbing, thinking, boycriedwolf's slow decline bothering me, our steam train losing momentum ... then this idea popped into my head.

**The Steam Train Analogy**
Steel deck engine room
Boiler door swung open
Coal shovelled, raging fire
Chimney exhaust bellows steam
Charging mountain, hugging iron
Determined face, dust-blackened

> Spotters peer open windows
> Rushing cool air collides
> Rotating wheels lose momentum
> Fuel stifles, revive fails
> Carriage emptied, disappointed passengers.

But really, this letdown was just another example of how minute my whole world had become. boycriedwolf's long, winding road to the end had left me feeling stranded on the platform of life while everyone else was on the fast train to getting on with it. Not on the steam train, because that ran out of steam—just a regular train.

I had put all my worth into boycriedwolf, underpinning my life's purpose to a band—*This was my only chance to make something of myself*—so strongly that I lost sight of the other members. The people who were doing this project, despite how much they loved it, for a little fun outside of their daily lives, jobs, school and families. It wasn't until a regular counselling session with the captain, where she said, 'Things sometimes just run their natural course and come to an end,' that it dawned on me that I was being a bit of a prune.

'You know what I'd like to do? I'd like to write about my stroke experience.'

'Well, then write,' she replied.

'But I don't know how. Where do I begin?'

'Just write. You write songs—just get it down on paper.'

So, with my one good hand, stretching my fingers across the keyboard—*F and C are just above each other, and the K is only four keys to the right*—I wrote, then I wrote, and then I wrote some more.

I couldn't stop. Words flowed from me like a burst water main, effortlessly, gushing out uncontrollably, sentences and paragraphs spilling everywhere, ankle-deep. Within a few short weeks, I had seven glorious chapters. The beginnings—thousands and thousands and thousands of tiny little letters, one after the other, spelling out words, telling my stroke story. *The U just above the K. Easy!*

While the librarian scanned my books, I saw a flyer sitting on the counter. 'Creative Writing Group—Members Wanted'. I grabbed my books and slipped a flyer in between one of the pages.

*A Week Later*
'Hey, everyone, this is Antonio. He'll be sitting in on our meeting today.'

Little did I know, these kinds of groups readily existed—apparently, you can find a creative writing group operating from most libraries! Super helpful for novice writers in need of a little guidance.

It seemed just perfect, exactly what I needed. A new purpose—*I often thought about writing stories, and now I had my own real-life tale to tell.*

I emailed the group my first submission, chapter one. *Oh, they're gonna love this.* Why wouldn't they? I had a cracking story on my 1.33333 hands—Vietnam, stroke, recovery, boycriedwolf—*It's gonna blow em away,* I thought. I was quietly confident, patiently waiting for our next meeting, anticipating pats on backs, handshakes—*Your story's amazing!*—hugs.

Now, upon reading the last twenty-one chapters, you may have concluded—at least I certainly hope so—that my storytelling isn't too bad. That I do okay spinning a yarn, and if you have a copy of this book in your hands, then it's likely a publisher agreed with you and decided my story was worth putting to print.

However, the creative writing group didn't necessarily see it that way. 'Take a little break from writing your memoir,' they suggested. 'Maybe write some short stories and submit those. Try and find your own voice, how you want to tell your story. Oh, and read a lot! It'll help you develop the skill of writing.'

After I finished plotting how I was going to assassinate each and every member, I took my not-so-favourable critiques—*Are these people mad?!*—home to readdress whether this new purpose of mine was worth pursuing. And then, once my ego tired itself out and lowered its arms, I thought maybe I'd have a go at writing short stories, read a lot and find my voice.

July seventh, 3:00 a.m., the morning after Charlotte and Molly's birthday. Yes, much to their disappointment they share a birthday, three years apart. I decided to let my assassination plans slide, and instead I spent a few months developing the craft of writing. I worked on short stories and poems, along with lots of reading. 'Try and find your own voice,' they had said. I just had no idea how. *What do they mean? Where do I look?*

Normally I'm a solid sleeper, but in the wake of my girl's dual birthday, while no one else in the Southern Hemisphere was awake, my eyes sprung open. Perhaps I'd eaten too much cake, my kryptonite.

So, I gave up the insomnia battle and rolled out of bed, feet shoulder width apart, stretched, then Chaplined my way into the kitchen. I flicked on the light and the kettle and booted up my laptop, made myself a one-handed coffee, pulled my chair back at my desk, sat, rolled it forward, then opened a new Word document and began writing.

There must have been another burst water main, *words gushing out uncontrollably, sentences and paragraphs spilling everywhere,* this time knee-deep. I was at it for about three hours till everyone in the Southern Hemisphere began to wake, then I hit the last full stop, save, and went back to bed.

The sugar rush from that birthday cake, combined with a burst water main of words, resulted in no sleep that night. While most everyone else was commuting in rush-hour traffic to work, I once again rolled out of bed, did the feet thing, stretched, and Chaplined to the kitchen—light, kettle, laptop—to find exactly what I was looking for.

*Stroke! But you're so young*! It was all there: detail, dialogue, humour, even this bit—*Language warning! I don't often swear, but #@$%, after what I've been through ...*

My voice!

It just arrived, unannounced, at 3:00 a.m. one night on a sugar rush—*sitting silently in front of my laptop, I typed with my one good hand.* That typing frenzy was such a high, a dopamine rush. No wonder I couldn't sleep.

Those embarrassing writing attempts I had submitted to the group were horrible; now I could see what they meant. 'Try find your own voice'—*der, McFly*. Of course. Now I got it. Someone take those not-so-glorious seven chapters, print them off, then run them through a shredder.

Now I could write this thing, bash it out, get it down on paper.

TWENTY-THREE

# The Lion Tamers

'Tell them at the very beginning,' she said. 'Give them an opportunity to get to know the real you. Don't try and hide your stroke. Be raw! Your music is raw, your writing is raw, and that's what makes you stand out from all the rest. And if she's worth it, she'll see all I see in you, plus more. But if she doesn't, don't be discouraged. It's just the world sorting out the right person for you!'

I reckon that would have to be the single most beautiful piece of advice I have ever received.

'Wear your tragedies as armour, not shackles.' —Brenda Clark Hamilton.

My disability is now a part of me, who I am, and the only thing I can do is embrace it. While my self-acceptance had progressed further into this triathlon, *the gunshot sound of the starter's pistol* no longer ringing in my ears, the *kkkssshhh* sound still continued. As the kilometres clicked by, I discovered that the else-acceptance, acceptance by others, had two components to it.

Component one—how others accept you, how you're treated. Are you made to feel normal? Are you included?

Component two—your own acceptance of whether you feel included or not. Basically, not caring about what others think about your disability.

And there's no other better way to put this to the test than through dating.

Swipe left, swipe right was the new norm used for courtship, so I followed suit and gave it a go.

Weeks passed with varying degrees of success—and I use the term 'success' unenthusiastically. A match here, unmatch there, a few hellos, several non-replies, a quick chat, a disappearance, lots of messaging and lots of abrupt endings, or 'ghosting,' as its now referred to.

Online dating seemed less a community for courtship and more a battleground to erode your self-esteem. Brutal.

'Yeah, sure, I'm free tonight.' She and I matched early one afternoon, played messaging ping-pong for a few hours—*Seinfeld, Thai food, lazy Sundays*—then moved straight to a phone convo, deciding to waste no time and meet up that night for a date.

*Oh, man, I'm an idiot!* I had just a few hours to spare before we met. *I should have told her over the phone when I had the chance!* I began to panic, couldn't think straight. *I can't meet her without saying something.* I felt dishonest. *I have to tell her ... it's only fair.*

The thought of her first seeing me walk made me incredibly nervous. *And my eye—what will she think?* Keeping mute about the demon would send cortisol hurtling through my body, amplifying my C-3PO/Chaplin walking technique, and when I get anxious, my brain shuts down and stroke stands up. *I know—I'll text her.*

So, I sent three messages, a trilogy of an explanation.

Text 1: 'Hi, there's something I need to tell you.'

Text 2: 'I was born a woman!'

Text 3: 'Okay, I'm just messing with you. I'm a stroke survivor.'

Her reply: 'It's fine, don't worry, just be yourself. Thanks for telling me, see you later.'

It was a super-hot summer's night; we met mid-evening at a busy inner-city gelati bar. 'Would you like to sit outside?' I asked, ice creams held high as we pushed through swarms of people ordering gelati at the counter. We stepped outside into the warm air and sat at round tables, nestled beneath tall umbrellas.

Things progressed nicely. We chatted easily, laughed about our favourite *Seinfeld* scenes, talked about life, love, kids and whatever. 'It happened in Vietnam.' There wasn't a lot of discussion about the demon, though; she never really asked any questions. Maybe curiosity didn't get the better of her.

To each their own.

However, I do find the whole avoidance thing bizarre. Over the years, I've noticed most people are hesitant to bring it up. They kind of pretend it's not there, the big white elephant in the room. Even when I leave wide openings for them to ask—*'Sorry, mate, I can't make it next Tuesday, I've got a physio session in the morning,'* eluding to the point that my health needs TLC—they'll just sidestep what I've said and move on to something else. *'Dude, have you seen the property prices lately?'*

I get it with strangers—that's understandable, but when it's with people you know, it feels weird. You're there together, catching up, you may not have seen each other since before your stroke, and it's clear as day that something's NQR, that something has changed.

It's a year later, so you're well on your way into your recovery, living a post-stroke life. Sitting face-to-face, talking about all matters relating to being human—work, society, family, sports, property, politics, weather—and you're putting the bait out there, inviting them to take a bite, ask a question. Encroaching in the space is the large white elephant, overshadowing the two of you, standing there beside you, grinning, but regardless of how close it is, they decide to ignore its existence. *Weird.*

On another 'made to feel normal' occasion, at a large family gathering, I was standing in a circle of about eight people. One of them, a distant relative, went around the group asking each person what they now did for a living. *I work in a chemist. I'm a waitress. I do sales. I'm a cleaner* ... But when it got to my turn in the queue, they skipped past me and went straight to the person standing on my left.

I found that really odd. *Why didn't they ask me?* Perhaps they feared it was a sensitive subject or worried it was too personal, too painful to talk about. I don't think anyone else noticed; it wasn't so obvious. I was at the beginning of sensing people's behaviour around me. *Another chapter to this stroke journey,* feeling tiny nuances that normally slip below people's radar. It's the nucleus of component one—how others accept you!

It's not easy for me to *not* talk about the demon. He's part of my everyday life, and took up a huge chunk of it around that time. I couldn't simply put him aside, clock off and leave him at the office, not bring my work problems home.

I'd much prefer to get it out there, lay it out on the table, reveal my cards early and then let's get on with playing the next hand.

*To each their own.*

Back to the date—my ice cream was melting down my one good hand, which left me a bit stuck, in a bind, as my remaining .33333 of a hand didn't quite have the wiping-away-ice-cream skill down pat. Long Arm had missed this bit.

There I was on a first date, elbow-deep in ice cream, trying to play it cool, attempting to show this lady who I'd just met that I was all over this disability thing *like jam on toast*. Trying to make her feel assured that I wasn't a liability, that I wasn't a man who couldn't even wipe his own hands.

We'd been sitting for about fifteen minutes, having a nice time, eating gelati and pleasantly chatting. *So far, so good.*

I had my eye on the side door back into the gelati bar, the entrance near the bathrooms. *I'll quickly finish my ice cream, then go wash my hands.* It was dripping everywhere, *elbow-deep.*

The fifteen or so minutes of sitting still meant my affected left leg was going to need a little warm-up before it was ready to be involved in the standing and sidestepping process, not to mention navigating around and over chair legs, peoples' feet, and densely seated bodies, all whilst nursing an ice cream hand.

'Excuse me, I'm going to go to the bathroom and wash my hands.' I stood, pushed the chair back, stepped to my left, wobbled a little, tried to find my balance sweet spot, and then began weaving my way through the obstacle course, knocking into backs of chairs, clipping feet till I got to the side door. *It wasn't pretty.*

Feeling self-conscious—*Hope she didn't notice*—I entered the bathroom, washed my hands and returned to my date.

'Hey, I'm back.' I pulled the chair out from the table, stepped through and took a seat. As I lowered myself into the chair, I could feel the energy was different; the mood had changed.

From then on, for the remaining hour or so of the date, our conversation idled along. It had lost its smoothness, stopped and started, pit and pattered.

I drove home wondering, *Maybe my walk to the bathroom put her off!*

Component two still needs work—*basically, not caring about what others think about your disability.*

I never saw her again.

This time, I took my friend's advice—*'Tell them at the very beginning'*—and met my date at a local bar. I felt far more relaxed, at ease, confident. Our phone chat had gotten some of those hurdles out the way, laid them out on the table, my hand played early.

After a splendid evening filled with banter, physical contact, and a few drinks to lubricate the night, I did the gentlemanly thing and walked her to her car. I leant in close to give her a friendly hug but was delightfully met by her lips as she moved to kiss me right on the mouth, holding it for a few seconds, lingering, then pulling away. *Wow.*

'Good night. Thanks for a great evening.'

'Bye. Nice to meet you—talk soon.'

That 'talk soon' comment didn't quite happen as she said. A few days later, I reached out to say hello. She didn't reply.

*I don't get it ... she kissed me!* Curiosity got the better of me, left me wondering why, so I spoke to a mate about it. 'She probably thought it through and realised she wasn't comfortable dating someone with a disability.' That's a pretty up-front thing to say, but I appreciated his honesty, and it's exactly what I had been thinking.

We'd had a great evening together, and I sensed she was enjoying my company. There was some gentle physical contact, hand on arm, palm on wrist. We sat shoulder to shoulder, seated together, side by side, on a cushioned window bench. Close.

Once I thrashed it out with my up-front and honest mate, he agreed that she had perhaps gotten caught up in the energy of the date, enjoying our connection as much as I was. But then she got home and had a chance to come down from the high, back to ground zero, life's reality. Disability dating presumably didn't fit into her idea of romance, and so she'd decided 'ghosting' me was going to be the easiest way to deal with it.

Brutal.

'Hey, bro, I'm putting on an exhibition to display the photographic work of the kids who've attended the workshops,' said Ric. 'Why don't you put something together and perform?'

He's the dude who had often visited me after hours in rehab. *'I borrowed this white coat so security would think I'm a doctor'*— that guy, and his timing, far better than a *drunken drummer at a New Year's Eve party,* just so happened to coincide with the completion of writing the first of (little did I know) very many drafts of this book: *Saigon Siren*.

'Yeah, man, that would be cool. I'll ask a few muso mates to see if they're interested.'

It only took two phone calls, a couple of days, an old upright piano and three of us meeting at mine to jam on a few new song ideas that I'd concocted with my underdeveloped one-armed Billy Joel piano playing technique. And thus, the Lion Tamers were born.

*Feet shoulder width apart,* I pushed through my legs, *bent like a banana,* and raised myself off the mattress. I found my balance, then Chaplined my way through into the kitchen. *It's like a ball and chain.*

My 'The only thing predictable about stroke is, it's unpredictable' motto was living up to its reputation, adhering to the analogy. For no apparent reason—'cause that's how stroke plays, dirty—I woke feeling like rubbish, in the middle of a *heavy-duty wash cycle.*

As I normally do, I flicked on the kettle, then went over to my desk and wrote 'BALL AND CHAIN' diagonally across my diary—in capitals, 'cause it looks grammatically expressive. BALL AND CHAIN. See?

I had my coffee, did some stretching, slipped on a jacket, and headed out for a reluctant walk, hoping the fresh morning air would release the dirty demon's throttlehold.

No such luck.

Back indoors, in from the cold, I sat at the piano, ball and chain at my ankles. With my fingers on the keys, tinkering about one-handed, playing whatever, it just came out—words, music, music, words. 'Standing too close to the fire, with my ball and chain' came hand-delivered—in capitals, 'cause it sounds musically expressive. 'Desolate, stripped of desire, with my ball and chain,' a gift from the Melody Lord. 'Can't see clear of the rain, my ball and chain.' Who's the Melody Lord, you ask? 'Try make it through every day, I can't explain.'

Some may say I have too much time on my hands to make up nonsense like the Melody Lord. Maybe so, but time, that precious thing we all have so little of, was the hidden treasure concealed behind the challenge of my adversity, and if used correctly, it could be my silver lining. Willy Wonka's golden ticket.

As for the Melody Lord, he visits me at night while I'm asleep, coming down from Melody Heaven to hum melodies into my ear. My job, when I wake, is to take those melodies and turn them into songs.

I'm a Melody Messenger.

Most of the photography works were in black-and-white. Ric had them eclectically hung across the shopfront art space as part of his nonprofit organisation called 1 Camera 1000 Smiles, teaching kids in disadvantaged areas some fundamental photography skills.

It was his own little baby, giving back to the community. The workshops stretched as far as Indonesia and the Northern Territory, and of more recent times, refugees from all corners of the globe living here in Melbourne. Considering it was a midweek evening event, a decent crowd turned up to support the worthy cause.

With an infectious positive energy, Ric worked the room, topping up champagne glasses, talking up photographs. A casual glance and a cheery nod our way as the Tamers performed a short acoustic set, low-key and intimate, of all original songs. A handful of pre-stroke tunes and the newly penned, first-time-performed 'Ball and Chain,' standard casing ... 'cause that's just the way it was.

And though performing wasn't necessarily on my list of things I wanted to achieve, I was on such a high that night, so thrilled. We all were, so much so that we decided to keep making music together.

'Let's record some songs, see what happens!'

Meetups at mine became a weekly ritual every Tuesday evening. The three of us, two acoustic guitars, the old upright piano, and my Tamer brothers' voices, workshopping ideas (Tamerfying), turning the Melody Lord's newly delivered melodies into songs.

I must have been Messenger of the Month the way I was absorbing those hummed hymns floating through me as I slept, transforming them into something new. Most mornings I'd get straight to work: wake up, *feet shoulder width apart*, push through my legs, raise myself off the mattress, find my balance, then Chaplin my way through into the kitchen, relentlessly dragging the ball and chain, some days heavier than others. Flick on the kettle, coffee, sit at the piano, then attempt to convert the melodies into songs before they slipped away, forever gone.

Once I had something nutted out resembling a song, when feel-good Tuesday evening came round we'd get together, sit around the piano joined by two acoustic guitars and our voices, and lose ourselves in the music. Tamerfying.

And though enough time had now passed for me to restart work on the second draft of *Saigon Siren*, it didn't seem as urgent. I'd told myself I was taking a break—'Once you finish the first draft, put it aside for a while to detach yourself from the story,' advised the creative writing group, now on my side; that 3:00 a.m. post-dual-birthday burst-water-main writing frenzy had won them over. But with the frequency of the melodies coming through, delivered by the Lord, the idea of stopping that flow of creativity led me to telling myself, unconvincingly, *I'll work on the book in my spare time.*

Instead, I began to focus all my attention on discovering ways to make music again, further developing my one-armed Billy Joel technique, learning recording skills and absorbing production knowledge. I'd align myself with my thoughts, feelings and emotions, digging deeper than I ever had before. I began writing notes in my phone—lyrics, verses, choruses and all—and sharing more of myself, more of ourselves, life, people, pain and happiness, re-establishing myself as a songwriter again, my deepest love. And as that was all pleasantly unfolding, without my awareness, *Saigon Siren* slipped the ranks. It effectively got shelved, priority paused until further unknown notice.

Tapping into some of those darkest memories through my recovery provided a labyrinth of ideas, a *smorgasbord of emotions*. I'd be on high alert, waiting for something or someone to trigger a feeling, an inspiration. I started searching for words I could use, phrases that had meaning, and before I knew it, the songwriting alignment technique began to produce results. It was beginning to work!

During a conversation with a friend, I told him how I'd felt after the radiation treatment had let me down. 'It was like my head was gonna explode. The pins-and-needles pain was intense.'

'You've just got to believe that you will get better.' He had hope in his eyes.

The advice stuck, resonated. I made a note in my phone: *These pins and needles, talk about believing, when gravity gets you down.* The song just fell into my lap, practically wrote itself.

I'd be driving, thinking about the impact of the depression that was still undergoing management, likening it to an invisible wall. Then when I'd get home, I'd rush over to the piano, and voila! *I've been running, I've been hiding, I've been trying to climb, invisible walls.*

To keep it all consistent, in theme with the whole bigger picture, the Tamers' nicknames kind of invented themselves.

First up—wise, grounded, Tamers' voice of reason—was the Governor, also the guy who had performed at my fundraiser party. One of my brother-like buddies, he was on vocals, ukulele, bass, and guitars.

Next, the youngest member who was always busy playing in other bands, a multi-instrumentalist, was the Rockstar, sharing vocal, bass and guitar duties with Gov.

And that left me, the Scientist, responsible for songwriting, music production, and one-handed piano and keyboards.

My simple post-stroke home studio that was used to record *intervals*, the first boycriedwolf album, was slowly expanding, growing into a humble laboratory for musical invention, hence the Scientist guernsey. And as the Tamers' sessions trickled along, week after week, month after month, season after season, our collection of recorded songs mounted into an impressive body of work that amazed us all. 'Hey, man, how the hell do you write these songs?'

The Lord moves in mysterious ways.

To say the Tamers were a contemporary-sounding band would have as much truth in it as this well-known presidential admission: 'I did not have sexual relations ...' Okay, okay, just checking to see if you're paying attention.

We drew our influences from The Beatles, David Bowie, Radiohead, Soundgarden, Nirvana and everything in between, and though we embraced modern technology, it was mainly used as a recording and editing tool.

We set no deadline to make the album. 'Let's take as long as it takes,' said Gov, *wise, grounded, voice of reason*. And that's exactly what we did. We'd record, then rerecord and rerecord some more. Chop, change, change, chop, arrange, rearrange, and arrange. A slow version, a fast version, one with drums, one with no drums— *Alright, already, I get the idea!* All this to say, we took our time.

'Hey, I'm gonna convert my laundry into a recording sound booth. Whattaya reckon?' That was really more of a statement, rather than me seeking approval. I already had the ball in motion, the plans drawn.

On the other side of the laundry wall was my dining table pushed to one side, my meals area turned control room where all the recording gear sat. By using an old retro Tandy Electronics microphone as an intercom system, and a lot of head scratching, *three days later* ... we connected the two rooms together for communication.

*Houston, we have liftoff.*

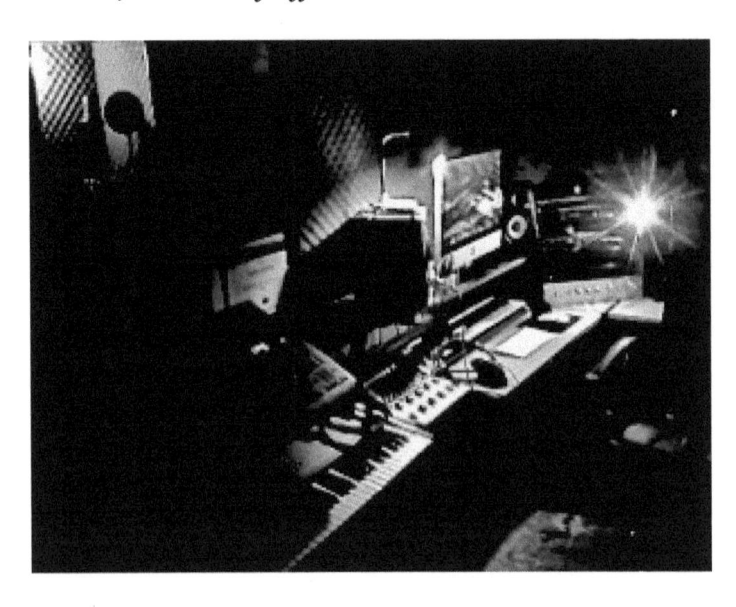

Still, I never really dealt with my depression. I tried to sweep it under the carpet, hoping it would just go away. Not even feel-good Tuesday prevented it from *rearing its ugly head*. Jamming with my Tamer brothers not a permanent remedy; the week was a mixed bag of all sorts. Miserable Mondays, terrific Tuesdays, wobbly Wednesdays, funky Thursdays, fantastic Fridays, Saturdays and Sundays just like the other ones.

'You're in denial,' said Doc Armstrong when I last saw him, but my resistance to his diagnosis wasn't based on not agreeing. I just wasn't so keen on using chemical intervention for my resurrection, and yet he didn't favour the organic approach. He was a science man, a NASA fan. 'Well, then, I can't help you!' Abruptly closing my medical file, fed up and frustrated, he suddenly made Buzz my new number one astronaut.

'You gotta take control, dude! What's the big deal? Just take the medication. If it's gonna make your life better, then just do it, man!' A good buddy had been called to come and rescue me. I was having the craziest panic attack, cortisol like a steam train hugging iron. Up until this point, all my other dances with anxiety seemed mild in comparison, scoring low with the panel of judges.

He pulled me aside and spoke calmly, 'Count down from one hundred by sevens,' attempting to distract me like SBS had when we'd circled the rehab halls.

'Dude, I can't even count down by sevens from seven,' I said, my thoughts scrambled, fried.

But distraction wasn't working. I was in such a state, reeling so hard—*my chest clenched tight, like I was biting the hose off during ICU phlegm suction.*

I'd never ever experienced anything like it. Honestly, it was frightening—scarier than that transition into the hydro pool, heavier than the angiograms, the radiation.

I needed help.

We took a casual ride over to the closest medical clinic, my buddy staying cool and collected, a bit like those paramedics who picked me up from the tarmac. After a short wait, we were able to see whichever doctor was next available to squeeze me in.

'Go easy on these.' He looked me square in the eyes. 'They're very addictive,' the doc said.

I'm not sure if that was the advice Elvis was given, but when anxiety came charging like a *Pamplona bull*, I swear I could hear those cute little moon-shaped pills calling my name. *Antonio, Antonio! Swallow one of me and the anxiety will let us be*!

Now, there's one little detail I haven't told you yet. It's the reason I flipped out and had a meltdown, and once you read it, you're gonna shake your head with dismay and say stuff under your breath like, 'Oh, Antonio, you ... !' I'll let you fill in the rest.

So, I was dating this woman for about three months. Yeah, I know, good for me, but steady on—just pause your excitement for a sec. It wasn't an overly serious relationship, and we weren't just FWB, either. Anyway, here's the missing piece of the puzzle. Are you sitting down?

She fell pregnant.

Bet ya didn't see that one coming.

Maybe you have less empathy for me now, cause the truth is, my own foolishness was the catalyst for the crazy panic attack. Self-inflicted.

The weeks that followed were spent attempting to handle the gripping anxiety, managed by moon-shaped pills as I tried to gaslight myself into believing that becoming a dad, once again, at the age of forty something, with a disability, was gonna be just dandy. *Maybe I'll finally get my son.*

It came as a complete shock, a surprise, putting our semi-serious new relationship into a much-too-early-to-deal-with difficult situation. Though we cared for each other, we weren't in love. It hadn't been long enough for that to have blossomed; we were still getting to know each other.

The pregnancy news soon filled her with joy. She saw this as an opportunity to finally have a child of her own, and immediately began making plans on how she would handle it, regardless of my involvement.

I had no idea how we were going to make it work. I was just barely managing to look after my girls, myself, my state of mind.

My self-gaslighting attempts seemed to have a gas leak. Some days, I warmed to the idea—*Oh, it'll be so cool to have a baby!*—and others I'd be stressing, turning to the moon to bring me back to Earth. *Self-inflicted.*

But I wasn't going to abandon her. That's not my style; I couldn't live with myself if I did. So, we began to discuss what was going to happen, how we would parent a newborn together, without us really talking about doing it as a couple. 'I'll be there for you,' I assured her, supporting her desire to become a mother while I wrapped my head around becoming a father ... of four.

But sadly, around the eighth-week mark, she had a miscarriage. It wasn't meant to be.

The stress from the whole pregnancy ordeal was coupled with continuing mixed-bag weeks: miserable Mondays, wobbly Wednesdays, funky Thursdays ...

Terrific Tuesdays quickly turned terrible, forcing us to take a short break from Tamers' ritual meet-ups at mine. The time had come to get off my organic bender and take my good buddy's advice—*'You gotta take control, dude! What's the big deal? Just take the medication!"*—along with Armstrong's science and a prescription from the Pilot.

Not using the mantra of 'ignorance is bliss' this time, I googled common side effects to expect and found disturbing comments left on forums. *Those pills made me grumpy ... They made me sleepy ... I felt dopey ...* Either those people had an unpleasant experience with medication, or a personal grudge against the Seven Dwarfs. Who knows?

Once the chemical intervention began, I couldn't distinguish between what were considered common side effects of starting anti-depressants—confusion, numbness, tingling, nausea—or the results of going cold turkey off the Valium. *Use them sparingly.* I only took them for about three weeks. *They're very addictive*—ain't that the truth.

Physical adjustment to having medication coursing through my system had a few bumps and potholes—insomnia, fatigue, dizziness, nausea—but it wasn't till one morning many, many months later that I knew I was back on track. I woke, went through the standard procedure—feet, stand, Chaplin, kettle, piano, sit down—and this fell out of me: *Say what's on your mind, leave the world behind and feel, so much better.*

The gluey taste of the stamp lingered on my tongue. I firmly pressed it to the CD mailer envelope, then joined the short queue before the counter. 'Next, please,' called the lady.

I stepped forward, said, 'Hello,' and handed her the envelope.

'Good morning.' She stuck the 'Delivery Guaranteed' sticker beside the destined address.

*That's our debut album in there,* I wanted to say. *We just spent the last two years working on it!* I was so proud, I wanted to let the whole post office know. *Attention, everyone! I had a stroke back in 2009, and a lot of the songs were inspired by it!* I'd say, nodding to myself, grinning.

She stamped the envelope, smiled and handed it back. 'Next, please.' I dropped it into the mailbox on the way out.

Mid-morning a day later, my phone rang. 'Hey, Antonio, I just got your CD, mate.' It was now in the hands of a trusted professional, ready for its final preparation: sonic balancing, known as mastering, the icing on the cake. 'I've had a quick listen to it in my car.' He sounded upbeat. 'The songs are great, the vocals are fantastic.'

My mind was blown. What a great way to kick-start your day—boosting your ego! In the thirty-odd years I'd been making music, that, hands down, would have to be the best feedback I had ever received.

No instruments were required for Tamers' next meet-up at mine; all that was left to do was design our CD artwork.

A few days prior, I saw this image in a magazine that caught my attention. It was made up of a series of small colourful squares creating a complete picture, and it kinda reminded me of the picture game the Duke and I had played during rehab.

'We should find an image for each song. Each image could represent something about the song.' We began Tamerfying the idea, applying the image concept to all the songs. We'd pick a lyric, a line, a feeling that mirrored each track's meaning while sitting around beside the piano, just as we did when workshopping melodies, losing ourselves.

'How about rolling dice for "Caramelized"?' It's the first track on the album, the opener, the lyric *'Choose your direction by the rolling dice'* appearing in the second verse. Just perfect.

Gov sat with a notepad perched on his lap, rough sketching, drawing concepts. 'We could use a skeleton for "Pins and Needles",' suggested Rockstar—*'These old bones can't stand alone'*—'and a brick wall for "Invisible Walls".'

It was all coming together, falling into our laps.

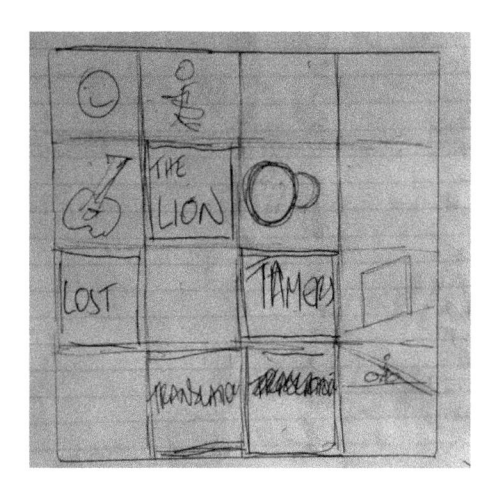

The eleven songs, shortlisted from a choice of fifteen, along with our band name and album title provided a perfect artistic layout for the album art. And you know all too well how I feel about balance—*as it has better symmetry that way.*

Two winters, a pair of springs, a couple of summers and a few autumns later, to the ecstatic joy of three awfully delighted dudes, *Lost Translation* was released.

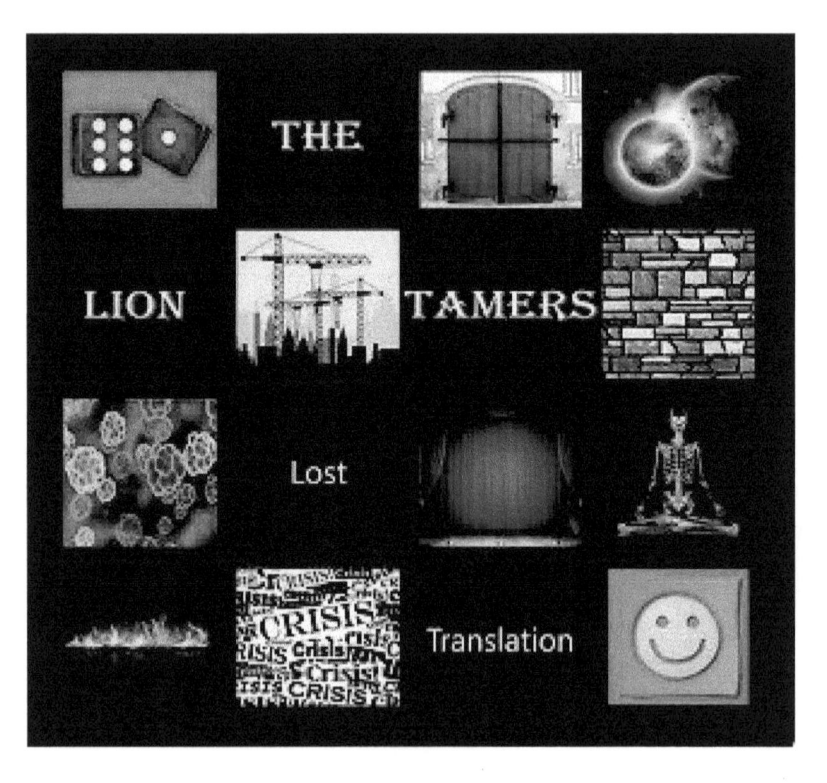

(Lost Translation album cover - Graphic Design by Emanuel Cachia.)

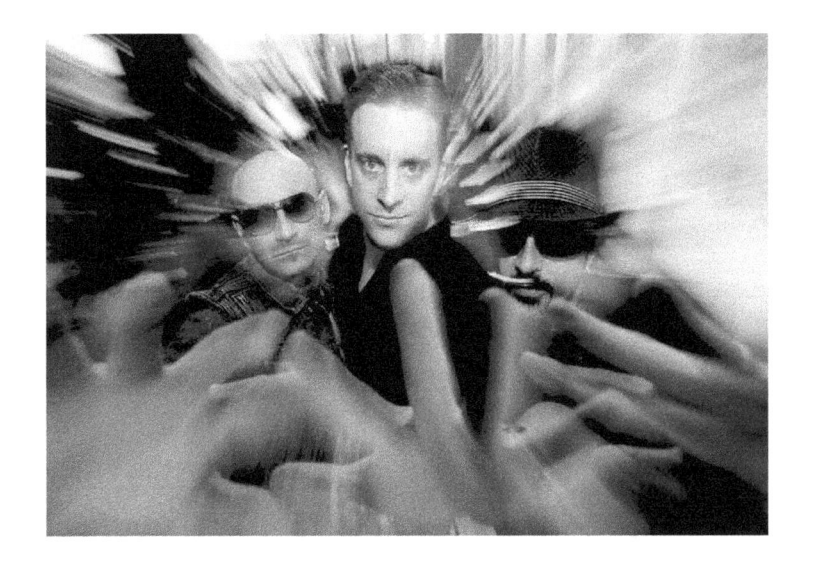

(The Lion Tamers; *L-R:* The Scientist, The Rockstar, The Governor
- Photograph by Ricardo Piscioneri)

TWENTY-FOUR

# Lucky

Have you flicked through to see how many pages are left to go? Heads up, it's fourteen, not including the acknowledgements. But who reads those anyhow!

Trust me, I'm just as pleased as you are to see the end. Writing this thing has been a mind-bender. There was so much to learn— *find your voice, write a few short stories, develop the skill of writing.*

Indirectly translating all that has happened into scenes, settings, legible stories and rewatching them all on my mind's *green screen* became my portal for personal growth. A place where I could journal the events, shred through the emotions, then rationalise their meanings, develop understanding, process it all and move forward.

Self-psychology.

Like the melting ice cream running down my arm on that date, when I was elbow-deep in the writing process it would be all over me, dripping everywhere, words, sentences, paragraphs consuming me. I'd go to bed thinking about it, wake up thinking about it, drive, eat, shower and sit *in the smallest room of the house* thinking about it. It kept me up at night and woke me early in the morning. My body would be dead fatigued, but my brain wouldn't switch off, at times causing a heated argument between them.

Body: 'Hey, you up there! Lights out—we're fatigued and need sleep!'

Brain: 'Shut up! I'm the master of this domain. We will sleep when I'm good and ready!'

I'd usually have to step in like an annoyed parent. 'Right, you two. Stop the bickering and get to sleep. Don't make me come in there!'

The creation of *Saigon Siren* was divided into two main periods, sliced in half by the Tamers project—pre- and post-.

Now, if you're thinking my mention of 'post-Tamers' is alluding to us breaking up, then you're spot-on. Sorry for dropping that news on you without a buildup or a wind down. We didn't dissolve like a keg of Palmolive Gold, after *Lost Translation* winning an ARIA, as I had imagined—*'And the best independent album goes to ... The Lion Tamers!'* Pity. I was looking forward to seeing Barnsey, thanking him for performing at my delusional homecoming street parade. Would have been good to catch up, have a beer together. *Saluti*.

It took two phone calls to kick-start the Tamers, but only one for it to end.

'Bud, you know I love the Tamers, but we can't go on like this. It's either in or out.'

Rockstar was keen to develop his own songwriting and release music as a solo artist, so when I sensed he was pulling away, I was a little ... well, shall we say, heartbroken. And after another no-show to a recording session of material for our follow-up album, yeah, I began to hold a grudge.

'Yeah, mate, I'm sorry. Life's pulling me in all directions at the moment. Let me think about it. I'll call you later.'

And just like that, The Lion Tamers ended.

*Pre-Tamers Period*

It first began when I had the novel—and naïve—idea to write a memoir. *Just get it down on paper*, they said, *then go back and edit it*. Sounds like good advice, hey?

After trying that, I discovered quite the contrary!

Learn the craft of writing first so the 'getting down on paper' part isn't a waste of paper and when you 'go back and edit it,' you're not doing your own head in trying to arrange eighty thousand words into an order that doesn't make you cringe and will provide some enjoyment for another person to read. This, I believe and have come to understand, through *firsthand experience*, is far better advice. Trust me!

But it's not uncommon for me to get an idea, then run with it like a horse with blinkers on, galloping to the finish line—'*I eagerly began writing about my experience in the shape of a book. When I arrived at thirty thousand words, I came to a grinding halt.*' Remember that?

'Once it's finished, give yourself time and distance from the book in order to untangle your emotional connection to the story,' my writer mates said. 'This will give you an objective perspective. Then you can commence drafting.'

So, I eventually arrived at the so-called 'finished book' finish line. I'd collected all the burst water mains of words into what I believed was a sensible order that told my story in a dynamic, heartfelt, and interesting fashion, along with all the frilly bits I've mentioned—*Stroke? But you're so young!*

The first opportunity, circa 2012, to potentially turn my new purpose into reality—to become an author, a writer—was at an event called 'Literary Speed Dating'. It was a crazy night, buzzing with emerging writers pitching their stories to a room full of Australia's finest publishers. Each writer had three minutes to bedazzle a publisher with a fancy spiel about their book. At the end of the three minutes, a buzzer sounded and you moved on to another publisher, just like speed dating.

And though the five publishers I spoke to all loved my enthusiasm—'*Wow, what a powerful story!*'—once I sent them *the so-called 'finished book,'* it was met with the same scepticism I'd gotten from the creative writing groups, pre winning them over. But all that enthusiasm only resulted in morale-deflating rejections once they saw the actual book—*'Thanks, but no thanks. Perhaps it could benefit from drafting. It's not what we're looking for.'*—giving *Saigon Siren* a helping hand to slip the ranks.

Cue the Tamers about here.

Once the Melody Lord began teleporting down from Melody Heaven to deliver his raw tunes, I didn't want to let him down; I feared he'd call in the Melody Mafia to come sort me out! And as those sweet hymns hummed in the dead of the night evolved into songs, the whole book idea slipped further and further, deeper and deeper, into the 'one day I'm gonna finish it' abyss.

*Post-Tamers Period*

There were a host of reasons, excuses, to prolong starting the second draft process. I buttered over my battered book dream's ego with distractions—counting backwards by sevens, working on side projects, producing music for other artists, family stuff, raising teenagers, cats in the cradlin'.

*I know, I'll break the book down into a collection of short stories!* I loosely ran with that idea for a while, trying to use the pandemic-induced downtime to tackle the enormous task and turn the virus that changed humanity into an advantage.

But Covid resisted, not keen to become a benefit. It stuck around far longer than we all anticipated, turning most people's brains to mush.

'One day, I'm gonna ...' I kept telling myself, believing my own BS, saying stuff like that just to feel better, to soften the realism of 'One day, I just may never!' It's a truth we all hate to face, denying ourselves the benefits that come with stepping outside of our knowns, our comforts, and instead surrendering to being too busy, too tired, unmotivated, consumed by lizardry—*flat-out-like-a-lizard drinking*. Then another day passes. Another week's gone. An entire year flies by. Pretty soon, ten years have passed, and you're no closer to achieving your goals.

That's exactly what I was doing: drifting.

Then, there was a turnaround. It came in the shape of a lady—*it's always because of a lady*. I was a little smitten by her. Well … maybe a *lot* smitten. She saw right through my disability, looking straight into my heart.

We met the standard way, online, and I kind of had a crush on her immediately when she asked—straight up, no BS—about my stroke.

I'd taken my friend's suggestion to 'tell them at the very beginning' one step further and added it to my dating profile, and as you can likely imagine, most people I chatted to online did the 'avoidance' thing. Even though it was there, in black-and-white—'I'm a stroke survivor'—no one dared to ask about it. Bizarre.

But not this lady. In fact, it was in her very first message to me. She mentioned her stroke survivor friend—spoke about how amazing she was, overcoming her challenges to rebuild her life—and I adored that about her. It softened me; my guard was down instantly.

So, by now you've probably worked out that I'm not very good at concealing my emotions. I'm more of a 'wear your heart on your sleeve' kind of guy, and as the weeks unfolded, during the very lovely getting-to-know-each-other phase, discovering our mutual passions—nature, art, music, writing—with my guard down and my heart open, I wrote her this poem.

Mind you, we hadn't met in person yet. At that stage we were only speaking a few times a week over the phone, just taking things slow. But I had this vision of her like I understood who she was, felt her gentleness.

Here's the poem.

*She wakes early to see the sunrise,*
*Puts one foot in front of the other and walks the sleeping hills through surrendering countryside.*
*'It's beautiful,' she says. 'You can hear the frogs. They're at their happiest.'*

*She stands magnificent, silhouetted by the early morning sun.*
*Words as soft as marshmallows gently wrapped in a thousand years of sincerity, tumbling from her lips, cascading from her heart.*
*I am mesmerised.*
*Paint upon paper, paper beneath paint, colours so pure you have to look away, hue so deep you forget to breathe.*
*With my eyes closed I can see her swaying, softly spinning, lost in rhythm, timeless, music moves through her, she loves to dance.*
*Her light divides the darkness, carrying me forward, beyond all I've ever known.*
*The place I long to be.*

The poem could have easily gone two ways, and for about three days I sat on it, considering the consequences, mulling it over. *She'll probably think I'm a creep*—that's one of the ways it could have gone. *We haven't even met in person yet.*

It was strange. I hadn't felt so drawn to anyone for such a long time. After a failed marriage and those dismal prior dating attempts, I began to concede that my life worked best being single.

The whole recovery journey of working towards personal growth came unconsciously coupled with me finally feeling, for the first time in my entire life, like a whole person—complete. And what I found was I didn't feel lonely; I didn't want a partner to fill any gap, but rather to be with someone where we could complement each other in a loving, nurturing way.

Sure, there are times I feel alone, and when I'm in a 'The only thing predictable about stroke is, it's unpredictable' state of mind, my resilience may be compromised and the feeling of loneliness creeps in. Then for a few days, maybe a week, my spirit is shaken and I'm reaching out to the people I love, my friends and family, for support.

What follows, with gentle encouragement and the handy personal growth tools I've accumulated along this endless triathlon, is a true sense of gratitude. An honest appreciation for life, a love for nature, the sun, the Earth, the trees, the air and the people, and soon my wholeness is complete again.

And for some reason, there was a knowing inside me. I felt that this lady was completely aligned with all that—*she gets it*. So, I took a chance and sent her the poem.

That knowing, the intuition, a feeling, touched her heart. She loved the poem, and we began dating.

Now for the turnaround bit. It didn't happen overnight; it was a gradual development. First it began with me telling her about *Saigon Siren*—'One day, I'm gonna ...'—trying to get her to believe the fallacy I told myself.

But she wasn't just gonna simply buy into my description of this alleged manuscript masterpiece that I'd been working on for too many years. She wanted to read it for herself, to determine whether my 'One day, I'm gonna ...' belief should remain exactly that—*one day, maybe, perhaps*. So, to give her a taste, I emailed her the first five chapters.

'It's so intense.' She had tears in her eyes. 'How frightening.' This was the turnaround taking place, in *real time*. 'And your girls ... so scary.'

That feedback from someone I cared about, who didn't sugarcoat the truth, who said it how it was in a nice way, shifted my drifting in the direction it needed to go.

She became my inspiration, my new confidante, as solid as a rock.

Then the real fun began—and I don't know why we all call it 'the real fun,' because what we're really talking about here isn't fun. It's damn hard work!

I didn't know where to begin. *Start from the top? Jump in halfway? Go backwards?* So, I rolled the idea around for a few days, giving it room to breathe, waiting for my brain to become as excited as I was.

It resisted. *'Oh, do I have to? I'll start tomorrow. Looks like it's gonna rain today.'*

*'I can't believe it, you're so lazy! Don't you want to finish it? You've been bragging about this book for ages!'*

'Yeah, but ...'

*'No buts, just get on with it.'* I put my foot down. *'Here's a suggestion: how about you start by taking a few days to read the whole thing, see how it feels?'*

'All of it?'

*'Yes, all of it! You're lucky you're not detachable!'*

Wouldn't life be simpler if we all could detach our brains for a while, even if it's only for a few hours a day, and give us a break from the incessant thinking? *Der, Antonio, have you not heard of mindfulness?* Yes, I have, and I practise it daily. But I mean us having an on/off switch, an ability to disconnect from our surroundings when things get too hard to deal with. The option to operate on autopilot till you're out of present danger.

After forcefully insisting my brain take a few days to read it through, *all of it,* I could see what the speed dating publishers were talking about—*Perhaps it could benefit from redrafting*—and was able to finally accept rejection. Not defeat, just rejection.

Once I recovered from how sick in the stomach I felt from seeing all the work it needed—*the 'real fun'*—to prevent burnout, I decided to slowly begin by making bullet points of ideas in my phone that I could develop into stories, then I would insert them into the book where needed. It's the same strategy I use for songwriting; ideas tend to flow best for me when I'm away from the source. Not directly thinking about it leaves the creative part of the brain to wander free, venture uninhibited.

The delusional homecoming street parade scene, the Melody Lord idea, the tofu theory ... all of those were conceived while I was away from the story. And though I've wished for many of the other misfortunes—the diaper explosion, salami dangling and Ruckman sponging—to have only happened in my imagination, they didn't. I've been scarred for life.

'You've got to finish it!' she'd say as I informed her about my writing progress. 'People want to read stories like yours. They'll get so much out of it.' She went about offering advice, support, suggestions. 'You should give your stroke a name.'

'Great idea, I'll think about it.' The next day, I texted her, 'How about Vaughn?'

Once my body and brain stopped bickering and joined forces, we finally got to the 'real fun'. There was another round of burst water mains, and soon words began to surge forth like a tsunami. I had new sections, rewritten chapters, scenes, settings, stories—more than I needed. I even went back through the whole overthinking thing again—*I'd go to bed thinking about it, wake up thinking about it, drive, eat, shower and sit in the smallest room of the house thinking about it.*

A newfound energy began to arise. 'One day, I'm gonna ...' turned into 'Now I will! I must! I have to!' I made a commitment to myself to work on the book each and every day. Even if I was having one of my 'The only thing predictable about stroke ...' days, I still honoured my commitment by, at the very least, doing something to move things forward, *anything*. It might be rereading a section, giving it a tweak, a quick edit—whatever. 'Chip, chip, chip,' she'd say. *My confidante, rock solid,* always wanting to hear about the details, the expression, the energy.

'You don't have to be great to get started, but you have to get started to be great.'—Zig Ziglar.

Setting targets and goals became a valued ally—*I'm gonna finish this chapter by Friday*—then I'd reward myself when I hit the target. When I achieved the goal, I'd treat myself to coffee, lunch, dinner, nature walks—a small acknowledgement, enough to celebrate the milestone as I ticked it off the list.

As this mindset grew, it spilt over into everything, I adopted healthier approaches to life, living, nutrition and exercise. Using the simple and so very affective goal-setting technique, I took it as far as writing a list in the Notes app on my phone of things I wanted to achieve, then marking them off when completed with a large green tick emoji. Then I would leave the item on the list with the green tick beside it instead of deleting it so that each time I visited the list, I would see the green tick, giving me an extra sense of accomplishment.

I began to feel my self-esteem vibrate at a higher level, a confidence that enabled me to reframe those rejections, appreciate the criticism and use them as a source to improve, as fuel to get better at my craft. To not give up.

Failure is a friend disguised as fear.

Small habits are not small at all; in fact, they're the stepping-stone to a greater vision. When we set goals, no matter their size, once we achieve them, the reward centre of our brain releases feel-good chemicals such as dopamine, adrenaline, oxytocin and serotonin, eliciting positive emotions to help us conquer our challenges.

I consider this to be the underlying factor of the whole 'law of attraction' theory. Healthy habits, applied to all aspects of life, align us with a higher frequency, a greater energy, and that is when we begin to attract what we desire.

It was Einstein who said, 'Everything is energy and that is all there is to it. Match the frequency of the reality you want, and you cannot help but get that reality. It can be no other way. This is not philosophy. This is physics.'

All things beyond the natural world, all things that have been created by human beings, began as a thought, an energy. Someone imagined it before it became reality.

When the telephone was invented in 1876, it began as an idea by Alexander Graham Bell. Then, over a hundred-plus years, through a journey of imagination, positive belief and, of course, *the 'real fun,'* that idea was further developed to become the single most obtained devise on the planet: the mobile phone.

Before the Wright brothers first took flight, they imagined the aeroplane. Then, with an unwithering belief, a knowing that it could be made possible, their imagination expanded into form—on December 17, 1903, Orville Wright piloted the first powered aeroplane twenty feet above a North Carolina beach.

We have to believe it before we can see it.

At the beginning, during the earlier days of my recovery, I had no idea how I was going to walk again. I was in such a desperate state, I just couldn't see it happening; I didn't believe. But slowly, as the light grew brighter and hope drew closer, I began to set my sight *on the grand prize: walking*. And with the Goddess's genius, focusing on small goals—*butt shifting, slow dancing, half stands, bent bananas*—each time I accomplished the goal or hit the target, without my awareness, the reward centre of my brain released those feel-good chemicals, providing me with the energy and positive belief to overcome the challenges.

What you think, so shall you become.

But, having said all that—and considering that some may find the whole 'law of attraction' thing a bit too New Age—I'd just like to clarify on some points about how positive believing, law of attraction and higher energies can be misconstrued.

Thinking positively won't win you the lottery. Aligning your frequencies will not automatically make you rich. Higher energy doesn't produce fortunes, solve all your problems or make you happy and healthy …

But what that mindset *will* give you is the ability to maintain the discipline required to turn the setbacks into kickbacks. Energy attracts like energy.

And to quote Zig Ziglar one more time, 'Positive thinking will let you do everything better than negative thinking will!'

I hope you're not too disappointed that I didn't ride off into the sunset on horseback with my lovely lady, living happily ever after. In the end, we decided to remove the romantic component out of our relationship and put our admiration for each other into being good friends. 'Sometimes the shortest relationships are the best ones we ever have,' she said.

While I was getting wasted on words writing this book, waking with rotten sentence hangovers, paragraph pain, full stop fever, I had a few revelations, epiphanies.

Without too much thought, no preconceptions, a handful of words rolled off my lips effortlessly. It was the most profound, unintentional thing I've ever said.

But I'll get to that in a sec.

I was now doing some volunteer work as a StrokeSafe ambassador for the National Stroke Foundation of Australia (NSF), raising stroke awareness amongst the community via public speaking presentations.

How ironic, hey? My self-appointed good deed position whilst in rehab, advising others about what a stroke really was—well, that fictitious gig flourished into real-life voluntary employment. Crazy.

If you've ever seen this campaign, FAST—an acronym for face, arm, speech, time—can be used to determine if someone is potentially having a stroke by following these simple steps. Starting with *F*, check to see if there's any drooping to the face. Then *A*, raise the arm, test if there's any weakness, movement or strength. *S* is for speech—can they speak? Are they slurring words? And finally, the most critical letter, *T* for time: acting quickly to call 000 just may save a life.

Spreading the FAST information was us stroke ambassadors' jam, bringing it to the people.

That unintentional 'words rolling off the lips' epiphany actually happened at an NSF stroke awareness presentation. Afterwards, whilst chatting to the organiser, she mentioned that her cousin recently had suffered a massive stroke and was struggling with her deficits.

'She's finding it hard to stay positive.' I certainly felt for her. 'The treating doctor advised us that the window for recovery was within a two-year period.'

I couldn't believe what I'd just heard. It wound me up. *Far out—that's what they told me.*

Given the new research about neuroplasticity (the brain rewiring itself after damage) that I was able to easily obtain and read about—and I know I'm no doctor—I just couldn't understand why a medical professional working in the field of neurology would be giving that disheartening advice.

So, I advised that lady, fulfilling my StrokeSafe duties, to reassure her cousin that the two-year window theory isn't exactly accurate. 'And tell her that life can be good after stroke.'

Now, this is the bit that just rolled off my lips without too much thought—the revelation. Straight after saying, 'Life can be good after stroke,' I said, 'If I had made a full recovery, I would have returned to my previous life, and I wouldn't have had the opportunity to experience all that I have!'

I didn't think much of it; I'd said it casually, trying to give her cousin some hope. It wasn't till later, when I was quietly chilling at home, that its meaning truly dawned on me. I swear, I was sitting on the couch thinking about the conversation and it just hit me like a steam train—*OMFG!*

It was just there, charging its way through, *hugging iron,* staring me blank in the face. It had taken forever to get to this place, after traversing through so many hurdles, trip hazards, roadblocks. Throughout most of the journey, my entire vision had been fixated on making a full recovery—getting to the final destination. And while I was venturing down new pathways, confronting challenges, rebuilding a new life, the reconstruction of a new existence morphed into something far beyond anything I could have ever imagined.

Vaughn had gate-crashed my life, muscled his way in and destroyed most of my possessions, trashed my soul. But what he couldn't break was that tiny little spirit that was flickering away deep down inside me, inside all of us. Even though at times I felt completely defeated—*Sometimes I wish I had just died on that day*—something that I can't explain just wouldn't allow me to give up.

Maybe it was my girls. I had to do it for them—they needed me. Perhaps it was my family, my friends, their love and support, or those kind strangers—*the incredible strength of human kindness*—that kept me fighting.

I don't really know what it was. All I know is that Vaughn isn't such a bad bloke after all. In fact, he has given me so much more than what was taken, often leaving me to feel like this is the happiest I've ever been in my entire life.

'Your stroke saved your life!' said a wise old friend.

And maybe, just maybe, through this whole crazy trip, the doctors were right. Maybe they actually knew what they were talking about, casually dropping the *L* word, slotting it into a sentence—*like a gold coin into a shopping trolley*.

'You're very … Mr. Iannella,' always said with good intent, with hopefulness.

And as the metamorphosis of my new existence took shape, carefully constructed from the 'greatest hits' of a previous life, those few words that I had grappled with believing steadily transformed, like a caterpillar to a butterfly.

'I'm *lucky!*'

## ACKNOWLEDGEMENTS

I am immensely grateful for all the wonderful support I received through my recovery—*the incredible strengths of human kindness.*

Through the writing of my memoir, to piece it altogether. I've had to frequently revisit all the painful events of my stroke. And now here I am, at the end of this decade long writing journey, taking a quiet moment to run it all through my head again, with the intention to thank those who were there for me. This time, I'm looking at it from a different perspective. I'm seeing myself completely helpless, hovering over everyone and watching them lose their minds doing what they can to save my life. And yes, once again, I'm writing this with tears in my eyes.

Though these words may only reflect a small fragment of the gratitude I have in my heart for all those wonderful people, many of them strangers. But here in these next few pages I'd like to express my love and appreciation for all the support I've received over the years.

That morning, at the tunnels, in the space of a few minutes, my life was turned on its head. It hurts me to imagine how frightened those around me felt, the panic, the fear and stress. I'd like to acknowledge my girls' mother, Silvia Tomarchio, for her incredible strength and courage during that crazy ordeal. And though our lives have taken separate paths, I'm thankful for all she did to get me home.

My daughters, Charlotte, Molly and Madeleine, have been my inspiration through my entire life as a parent, pre and post stroke.

I never imagined I could love someone as much as I love these three young ladies. Thank you for all the love and affection, all the help through the difficult times, stepping up to do those tasks that are beyond my stroke affected ability, and for just being beautiful human beings. I'm so proud.

Once I arrived back in Melbourne, I longed to see my family. Having them there every step of the way was the love I needed to keep me afloat. They were my foundation. My Dad Rosario, sisters Angela and Carmel, I love you all so much. And my brother Remo, your enormous support, there by my side in ICU, it gave me hope, love you bro.

It broke all our hearts when our beautiful mum Lina suddenly passed away. I take comfort in knowing she's watching over us all, her heart full of joy. Proud to see us looking out for each other. Love you, miss you.

Many of my close friends displayed heartwarming care through my recovery. My great mate Ricardo Piscioneri, Ric, the guy who would sneak into the hospital outside of visiting hours. We've been best friends for close to thirty years. He's someone I turn to often, speak to almost daily. He's been a solid soundboard through my years as a disabled person, offering help, advice, feedback on my creative pursuits, conducting photoshoots, building a website, fixing a sticky door ... He never received a nickname through the book. But I often refer to him as MacGyver. Thanks bro, love you man.

Mario 'The Governor' Ortega, he's like the older brother I never had. Our friendship began in 1995 as The Braves, an acoustic duo. We performed across Melbourne, making a living as musicians. Mars was like a mentor to me. His friendship I cherish deeply. Thanks for being there bro, love you heaps.

Heather Tutwiler, probably the only person on the planet who I can talk to about absolutely anything and everything for hours and hours. Always there to listen, always around to hear. A woman with the biggest heart and smartest mind, a great combination. Thank you, Heather, for being you, love you so much.

I've only known Penny Wong for about four years. But she's been a great friend, referring to me as her brother. So sweet. I was overwhelmed with gratitude for the way she cared for me during a medical procedure I had mid 2024. Thank you my dear.

During my post stroke life there has been many people who I grew close to. Some of those I saw frequently during certain periods of time, some came and went and some I may not see often but know we have a forever connection. Thank you.

Chris 'The Rockstar' Williams. That Tamers period, making music, hanging out, conversations, learning, growing, supporting, is a time a hold dearly. Thanks for believing in me.

Alexa Banks, I've not seen her in over twenty years; haven't been able to make it back to London. But I wanted to send her a huge thanks for pushing me to write better. Your critiques of my chapters inspired me to dig deeper. Nice one.

Trace Balla, the catalyst for the turnaround. Thank you for believing in my story, my writing, my creativity and for giving me that nudge to get it finished. It probably would have remained, *'One day I'm gonna,'* if it weren't for her.

Emma Spiteri, thanks for your friendship, the conversations, the caring advice, feedback on my writing ideas.

A special thank you to a man I only knew briefly, until he become a key figure in saving me on that daunting day. Chister Ho, Thanks for all you did, you're a true gentleman.

I huge thanks to the boycriedwolf team; Mark 'Round House to the Head' Nolasco, Ebony 'Young and Talented' Roach, Steve 'The Italian Stallion' Cannizzo, and an extra shout out to Adam 'Machine Man' Roach for joining me on my very first post stroke musical quest and the continuing, revived, boycriedwolf. Looking forward to releasing more music together.

My rehab team made me feel so safe, so cared for and so supported. Anna 'Rock Goddess' Mathews, Sharon 'Long Arm OT' Vella, Marlise 'Short but Sweet', Anna 'Diagram Lady', Anne 'Houdini, Grey 'Duke of Earl' Searle, Lee 'Captain' Simonds, S.P, Lauren

Farrugia, Trudy Westley, Dr Shepard Chifura, and my stroke buddy, Sarah 'Snow White'. Thank you all.

And a big thank you to the extended circle of people who visited, helped, cared, and supported. My large Italian family, nephews, nieces, brother and sister in-laws, uncles, aunties, and cousins. Through to the medical team, The Mechanic, Napoleon and wife, The French Revolution, Captain America, The Rowing Team, The Coxswain, Neil Armstrong, The Pilot, The Captain, Radioman. A special shout out to Sandra Lenzi Portaro, Julien Campbell, Denise B. And to my old work colleagues: Glenn, Sally, Scott, Joel, Tassie, Gerry, Marie, Carol and Ian. Cheers.

Craig Henderson, Emanuel Cachia, Terry Probert and The Wordsmiths. Thank you all for critiquing my early writing efforts, giving me direction, your honesty and helping me grow as a writer.

Through the final drafts and edits of my manuscript, the pointy end of the journey. Cleo Miele jumped on board to help fine tune my prose, punch my grammar into shape and offer some small, but oh so very helpful structural tweaks. Thanks Cleo, up till now you're the one and only person who has read my entire book.

A few years into my recovery I became a volunteer at the National Stroke Foundation of Australia (NSF). My role as a Stroke Safe ambassador was to primarily conduct stroke awareness presentations to community groups across Melbourne. I found this position extremely fulfilling and rewarding, being part of a kind and caring team of people provided me with an enormous sense of belonging. This short paragraph is dedicated to those passionate members of the NSF. Thank you for all your support and for all the wonderful work you do to help minimise the impact of stroke. You're the best!

And let's not forget Ainz Charlton and Urshabloom, for those amazing years of music making, the London gigs, rehearsals and recording sessions. Cheers dudes, so much fun.

Last but not least, to all those I met, the doctors, nurses, therapists, that Aussie guy and First-Aid nurse who helped drag me to the bus. A giant thanks to you all.

And one more thing, to you, the reader. If you've read these acknowledgments, then it's likely you've read my book. Thank you, I hope you've enjoyed it. I feel honoured and privileged to have shared it with you.

Much love, peace, health and happiness to everyone. Antonio

Milton Keynes UK
Ingram Content Group UK Ltd.
UKHW041946091024
449514UK00006B/43